A WOMAN'S CHOICE

Samuel J. Barr, M.D.,
with Dan Abelow

Rawson Associates Publishers, Inc.
New York

Library of Congress Cataloging in Publication Data

Barr, Samuel Jacob, 1934–
  A woman's choice.

  1. Abortion. 2. Abortion—Psychological aspects.
I. Abelow, Dan, joint author. II. Title.
HQ767.B28 1977   301   77–76995
ISBN 0–89256–025–8

Copyright © 1977 by Samuel J. Barr, M.D.,
with Dan Abelow
All rights reserved
Published simultaneously in Canada by
McClelland and Stewart, Ltd.
Manufactured in the United States of America
by The Book Press, Brattleboro, Vermont

Designed by Gene Siegel
Second Printing March 1978

To those who love and those who have
the warmth of understanding

To those who feel that needless pain
and death are not a virtue

To those who have the courage and
the will to make life better

ACKNOWLEDGMENTS

I would like to give thanks to

Dan Abelow, whose gentle hands molded my thoughts and words into the form of this book;

My publishers, the Rawsons, who had the courage to let me tell this story;

Joan McIntosh, whose tireless dedication to collecting information is enormously appreciated;

My staff, for their contributions and observations, most especially Harriet Wooten, Deborah Herchig, Dottie Hicks, Joy Jones, Clara Nell Ellixson, Betty Crocker, and Rita Bannister;

Marie-Louise McIntosh, for endless hours of transcribing and preparation of the manuscript;

And last but by no means least, my wife, Linny, and my children, Debbie, Lisa, and Kenny, who gave so many days and nights of their own rightful time to their Daddy's efforts to write this book.

CONTENTS

IV. WHERE ARE WE GOING?

FOREWORD

A Woman's Choice is an especially timely book. The choice of whether or not to continue pregnancy—so humanely universalized for American women by the Supreme Court in 1973—now stands in jeopardy of abridgment or nullification. Those who advocate such changes must be little aware either of the human anguish caused by an unwanted pregnancy or of the social and personal damage occasioned by forcing such a pregnancy to term.

It is the universality of this multifaceted problem to which this book speaks with sensitivity and with great empathy. Because of their very wide experience, the authors are able to let women of all ages tell their stories. Those who speak are not preconceived stereotypes whose problems have simple causes and solutions. They are real human beings. The causes of their unwanted pregnancies, the impact of these pregnancies, and the solutions to their many problems are as varied as their number. They could be you or a member of your family.

You may well be tempted to close this volume, once

you have read of these women and the stories they tell, without glancing at the Appendix. If such be the case, you will miss much factual data on both medical and political aspects of the abortion question. These data you should know, for we in the United States are now engaged in a debate on abortion issues, issues for which there are no simple answers. Further, it is impossible that all the people in this large and varied country will be satisfied with whatever answer is forthcoming. Dr. Barr and his co-author have clearly presented the very human and factual dimensions of the abortion issues. It is hoped that their intelligent presentation of the human facets of the problem, which are so often ignored or unknown, will help the people of this country make a wise decision about these vitally important, emotionally charged issues. The time for decision is not far off.

Louis M. Hellman, M.D.

I

WHO IS INVOLVED?

1
WHERE DO YOU FIT?

There are two timely topics I'd like to share with you, about which I have new things to tell. Both may touch your life, regardless of your daily interests, social standing, or personal philosophy. The first is not abortion, despite the fact that much of this book offers a landmark understanding of what it's all about. The first is an insight into today's changing world of women and men and an aspect of their attitudes and relationships from ages ten to fifty, which are so different from even a generation ago.

It is hard to realize, but it's only within the past hundred years that women have gained the right to choose *with whom* to have a family. At the turn of the century marriages were still largely arranged by parents. Many a bride and groom got to know each other, literally, on their wedding night.

It is less hard to realize, since it is within the memory of so many of us, that it is only within the last thirty years that women have gained the right to directly control *when* to have a family. At that time the successful development of

3

the birth control pill ushered in the Age of Contraception. Until then, contraception was a chancy thing, and often as not determined by the male.

And only within the past decade has the right of a woman to decide when *not* to accept a pregnancy—the right to abortion under certain conditions—been recognized. Most women and men view motherhood as a blessing, under even half-decent circumstances. But when these circumstances are intolerable, women no longer need feel themselves the helpless victims of biology.

At present, the right to determine *when never* to become pregnant is also in resolution. The reasonable availability of sterilization is becoming a wider possibility.

These developments are now phasing out thousands of years of social programming that quietly assumed that the only valuable function of a woman was to have and raise children. These are not simply side issues of women's liberation, and their benefits are not for women alone. The new freedoms in childbearing decisions and the right to self-identity inherent in these freedoms affect the personal rights of men and oncoming children as well.

Over a million women every year request abortion, the greatest majority of whom have the strong support of their husbands, lovers, and/or parents. The average abortion request touches the lives of at least six other people, including the foregoing, friends, physicians, ministers and other professional counselors. Since legalization, more than 30 million people may well have been involved. These astounding numbers existed before legalization as well.

Where do *you* fit?

The sheer number of those involved makes it likely that your life has already been touched by the problem in some way, whether you realize it or not. Even if you have not yet been involved, you very well may be. And if you understand more about this subject, you surely will have a new depth of insight and compassion for those involved.

Share with me what I've learned.

Several years and some twenty thousand cases ago, I opened a clinic called EPOC, which stands for Every Person's Own Choice. There were so many unmet needs. During that time I had the early opportunity to study real people with real problems. Their relationships and reactions, taken together, are a composite of the changing attitudes of today.

There are good reasons why the public's attitude toward abortion has evolved from one of censure to more open acceptance. The case that got me interested in abortion occurred while I was a resident in training in obstetrics and gynecology. At the time, we had special wards that often were filled with patients who had been admitted with a spectrum of pelvic disorders, which had resulted from infection and hemorrhage, following illegal abortions. I treated a number of these women during my term of service and spent many a long night and morning in surgery with the attending staff, working to keep these women alive and to preserve them as much as possible from winding up as pelvic cripples.

I'll never forget one patient; she was thirty-two years old and the mother of two children. She was admitted through the emergency room with only a moderate fever and blood in her urine. She wouldn't say anything except that she thought she ought to get help as soon as possible. Because she didn't have a private doctor, she came directly to our hospital.

Her symptoms were relatively mild. Her pelvis was moderately tender and her uterus was only slightly enlarged, but she did have a positive pregnancy test. There was one other finding: a small puncture point with a little bit of bleeding at the entrance of her uterus. All the laboratory and bacteriology studies were started. I suspected that either she had tried to abort herself or someone else had done it to her. When I checked on her a little later, I had to press the point of asking her what happened because she had visibly weakened.

"I had to do it," she said. "I went to this lady who put a coat hanger up in me. She told me not to panic but if there were some real problem, don't say anything but go to the emergency room. I figured that blood coming out whenever I went to the bathroom was a problem and I got real scared."

With luck, I thought, the worst diagnosis would be that this woman's bladder had been perforated. That would not be pleasant, but hopefully there wasn't any major systemic problem. I started massive antibiotic treatment immediately, beginning with several transfusions to replace the blood she had lost. I had been through similar cases and felt things would work out well.

Three hours later I learned I was wrong. Only minutes apart, two phone calls told me of her terrible fight to stay alive. First, the laboratory reported that preliminary studies indicated an infection with gas gangrene. Then, the nurse on the floor said that the patient looked just awful—she wasn't bleeding much but she had a lot of difficulty breathing. I ran to the floor and found her slipping rapidly into heart failure. The professor who headed our program came in to assist, but everything that twenty skilled people could contribute did not help. The gangrene bacteria were destroying her red blood cells. That vital fluid was turning into little more than red water. Her heart couldn't handle it and her body was dying. All the drugs, machines, and people who might help didn't matter. The last thing I remember her saying to me was, "I know you tried. Figure some way to tell my kids. They won't understand it all. Tell them for me somehow. I don't want them to think me bad." She lost consciousness then, and a little bit later, just before dawn, she died.

I was very depressed that day. The other doctors told me of many similar episodes they had seen, but that didn't help. I never did learn the reasons that led this woman to risk her life in an illegal abortion. Whatever the reasons were, I'm sure they were overwhelming and significant, at least to her. I knew that she had been trapped, that there had been a senseless, useless, stupid waste of a woman's life, that something was wrong, terribly wrong. The lack of the safe, easily available help that has become common today had caused a needless loss of a real woman, a real mother, a real human being who should not have died this way. I still remember and feel that loss as if it happened yesterday.

I confess that this irrevocably changed my thinking. I was shocked by this totally needless waste of life to the point where I felt that whenever abortion should become legal, as one day it must, I would do everything in my power to eliminate and prevent this kind of tragedy.

This book is part of what happened to me that day.

In my clinic I have learned the real needs for abortion, not just the requests. I have discovered why women have unwanted pregnancies despite the availability of birth control, broader sexual knowledge, and no lack of intelligence. I have learned that the increased search for self-identity has created both advantages and disturbing confusion in current relationships between teenage women and their parents, and adult women and their mates.

Thousands of patients have revealed the problems that can be caused by careless or frankly malicious professionals, and the pitfalls that can be avoided in seeking an abortion if one has a basic background of information. Even the circumstances under which to opt for adoption or for keeping a pregnancy have become more clear. With the passage of each month, I have come to realize more acutely the great preventive help that government could offer, and how many tragedies it has contributed instead.

The women I've met were not predominantly wild or promiscuous. The men who came with them were not simply anxious to get a guilty responsibility out of the way. Their reactions were strong but varied widely.

So far as teenagers go, when the courts declared that youngsters don't need parental consent for abortion, the newspapers and television resounded with horrified cries of anguish. "What! My daughter can do whatever she wants and there's nothing I can say about it?" In fact, there are very few problems along these lines. Most of the real difficulties turn out to be exactly the reverse, with frantic parents accompanying a thirteen-year-old who thought it would be nice to have a dolly of her own.

All these people break the molds, which never were real to begin with. They are a cross section of everybody, from the peaks of the social register to the depths of welfare, and every conceivable step in between. In my clinic alone they represent enough national origins to make up a pregnant United Nations. They are of all races and religions.

Where do *you* fit? If you are not too old to feel love and concern, then you fit in right here. Right here, with all the rest of us.

2

DO YOU KNOW THESE PEOPLE?

Women from every background share one thing in common: the possibility of an unacceptable pregnancy. Before legalization, approximately nine hundred thousand women a year faced an overwhelming personal crisis and had nowhere to turn. Hundreds of thousands of families each year had to deal with unwanted children brought into the world.

Back-door, frequently catastrophic abortions were the only escape from this trap. Surveys have shown that between 50 and 70 percent of all women with unwanted pregnancies risked their health at the hands of untrained butchers. Poor and rural women suffered most. They were least able to find even semiskilled practitioners. Frankly barbaric measures used by self-appointed abortionists jeopardized thousands of lives on a daily basis.

An unwanted pregnancy is no longer as difficult a situation because skilled medical and emotional care is available. The women who encounter this problem do not fit formulas. They vary greatly due to where they are in their life span.

To Age Eighteen: Early Sexual Capability Before the Formation of a Lifestyle. Today, a large percentage of young women under the age of eighteen are sexually active. This doesn't mean that they are promiscuous. Teenagers are not hopping in and out of bed with a variety of partners. But when little Linda has been going steady with Tommy for six months, it's time for mother to consider carefully that her little girl may not be much of a child anymore.

Who in this age group needs our services at the clinic? We see young women from all kinds of families and all kinds of backgrounds. We've seen not just one but more than two hundred youngsters of age nine! Add more in the ten- to thirteen-year-old group. The fourteen- to fifteen-year-olds are averaging half a dozen a week, which is about one unwanted pregnancy a day. And in the sixteen- to seventeen-year-old group they need our help by the thousands.

How do these young women feel about being sexually active? After their procedure most of them request birth control to prevent future pregnancies, and the method of choice is usually the pill.

Young women become pregnant mainly because of a lack of honest communication about needing contraception. It is a pathetic stroke of irony that fearing to upset parents leads teenagers to avoid making them accept their sexual maturity. Parents continue to pretend that teenage daughters are still children, and daughters allow them the continued pleasure of that illusion. Neither wants to shatter a comfortable image. Under these very frequent circumstances, the image is shattered indeed by an upsetting pregnancy. It might have melted more gracefully and been replaced by a stronger, certainly safer reality, if given the chance of honest confidence and a measure of respect going both ways.

At the age of fifteen, Natalie's physical development was the envy of most twenty-five-year-old women. She was a responsible youngster who neither looked nor acted like a child. She was not treated like a child, most especially by her boyfriends, and enjoyed all the attention and fun of feeling quite grown up. "I tried intercourse a couple of times a year ago," she said. "I guess it was all right. I mostly wanted to see what the fuss was all about, but I always felt that if that was all someone wanted, I could easily get another date. It just wasn't worth the hassle, so I didn't really need birth control.

"Everybody said my attitude was cool," she continued. "I know where it's at, and they treated me okay. Tommy, though, turned out to be different somehow, and it just sort of happened. Now I don't know what to do. There's just no way I can feel good about it.

"I told my parents and it upset them. They didn't scream or anything. They said that they had been afraid this might happen, but hoped it wouldn't. Mostly, they wanted to know how I felt. Right then, I didn't know. One of my friends said that they had pregnancy tests at a pro-life clinic, so I went there. They said I should have the baby and could adopt it out, but if I had it I'd want to keep it. But what happens then? I want to finish high school and my marks are good enough to go to college. Everyone always said that I should go if I can. It was terribly confusing but the clinic said it would all work out. I asked them how and they couldn't tell me. They suggested getting married, for a start.

"I tell you, I guess I could get married, but I don't really want to. Not now, and not to Tommy, the more I think about it. That sounds horrible and selfish, but I can't pretend and just keep pretending forever."

Natalie knew some girls who became pregnant in high school, then dropped out to get married and have the baby. For a while they were miniature celebrities. Then the admirers went back to their own lives, and the young mothers didn't feel popular and important anymore. They were too young and didn't have the money to be part of the adult world, and they were too tied to a baby and an apartment to be part of the high school crowd. Natalie didn't want that for herself—not one bit of it.

"I think I'd like to be a teacher," she said, "or maybe a nurse. I'm not really sure of exactly what but I want . . . I want that chance."

Cynthia, on the other hand, was not hesitant about young motherhood. By the time she finished seventh grade she never felt that her parents represented much more to her than people who fed her and told her what to do, most of which she'd rather not. She quickly tired of being treated like a child, and by the age of sixteen she was ready to make the break and run her own show. Larry, an eighteen-year-old, sensed this, won her confidence and the fun of playing with her blossoming little body by joining with her in downing her parents. With more selfishness than malice, he cheered on the normal rebelliousness of a teenager reaching for her own identity, and by hinting about marriage being the key to real freedom, cheered her right into bed.

When she became pregnant, Cynthia went into a panic. The cold chill of reality shot down her back. She couldn't go to her parents for a cozy warm chat about what might be best or not, because she felt it would amount to nothing more than another big hassle. She was not going to crawl on her belly just to be told again that she was an ungrateful, rotten kid. She decided to put it all on Larry. "You promised!" she cried. "You said we'd get married and it would be great. If you leave me like this I'll tell the world about it. We can live on what you make, and anyway, think of all the fun we can have at night. You always said you liked me better than anyone else you ever knew."

The happy couple drifted off into the sunset to start a marriage together, just like on TV, and with the same mixture of wishful thinking and fantasy.

For a while it did seem to work, but the rest of their story is the part that they never show after the last commercial. Cynthia had her first baby, then her second. She escaped from what she thought of as her parents' jail and found herself in a much smaller, less comfortable cell. Here, she couldn't even complain, because she set it up herself and, besides, it didn't do any good. Washing clothes every week and cooking every night weren't nearly as bad as cleaning up a baby's mess, and, dammit, she had to work just as hard when Larry had a day off. He turned into even more of a drag than her parents were. At least they didn't bitch, bitch, bitch that they were paying for it all. He finally took off for the hills, and at the ripe old age of nineteen, Cynthia showed up at the clinic. She looked a lot worse than an average forty-year-old, with her third pregnancy, no husband, two kids, and the doors slammed shut back home.

Our counselors wanted to say something encouraging, at least, but even they felt totally helpless. There was so little left to work with. It had all been used up too soon. "Hooray for welfare," Cynthia said. "Let's get on with it. Don't worry about a thing. I can manage just fine."

Another kind of adolescent confusion is seen in the clinic when a young woman of thirteen or fourteen is brought in by her frantic parents. "Mary Ann wants to keep her baby!" they cry. "*We're* not going to raise it. Doc, it's driving us crazy getting her to grow up halfway straight. She thinks having a baby is cute. *You* tell her something."

We've run into this kind of situation so often that we've come to call it the Dolly Dilemma. It is an ordeal for everyone involved. No one feels that any pregnant female should be badgered out of a pregnancy; this cuts off all trust and communication, precisely the qualities needed in counseling if a teenager is to be helped to develop a constructive lifestyle.

The only key is a delicate application of the firmness that comes from experience and an objective review of eye-opening realities. If this can be pursued with calm honesty rather than uncontrolled hostility, it sometimes has the chance to get through.

The questions that have to be raised are the real questions of formulating a personal future. How well can you do in school worrying about a baby too? Do you think your parents want to support you and the baby indefinitely? Are you prepared to live with David or Andy or whomever for the rest of your life even if you could get married? Don't you think that you'd like to have a good job and be independent someday? How would you feel if your twelve-year-old girlfriend was pregnant? What would you suggest to her, since you're older?

These are loaded questions, but they are not unfair. The difference between children and their parents is not so much one of intelligence as it is one of experience and the result of exposure to the realities that are the building blocks of life.

Hopefully, this young teenager will realize that adulthood is a state of self-sufficiency, which means being able to provide for herself and others. Keeping a pregnancy at too young an age does not help a woman develop self-sufficiency. In fact, it may prevent it and force a woman to be dependent on her family or a husband for the rest of her life.

Eighteen to Twenty-four: Sexual Maturity While a Life Pattern Is Forming. Ages eighteen to twenty-four mark one of the most important developments in a woman's life. As women in this age group describe it to us, the roles in which they find themselves expand to include being loved emotionally and physically, without severe threat to their identities, which they are actively forming. Being cared for does not restrict these women's independence or maturity. It is a warm, pleasant, and natural addition to their lives.

More than any other time in life, these years generally offer the greatest range of searching and experimenting with lifestyles and relationships, and probing to determine those that best fit each woman's unique needs. This search causes many changes in values, goals, associations, and lifetime priorities. As the mid-twenties are reached, by choice or chance the options leading to security or self-sufficiency are not restricted, but they do become more clearly defined.

After Emily graduated from high school, she entered a training program in a local hospital to become a medical technician. She was moderately interested in her work, but primarily seized the chance to escape the routine she found in her first job as a secretary. Sylvia, on the other hand, had a real artistic talent and a nimble ability with words. She took two years of courses in advertising, then began working at a top-flight local ad agency. Neither of these women ruled out getting married and having a family, but they felt no urgency about it. They enjoyed the freedom and pleasures of being able to earn a good living on their own. This took the pressure off any need to rush into marriage, and opened the door to active lives in which they met interesting people and grew rapidly. Even though

they both became pregnant, they reached the same conclusion as so many women in their generation: It would
be better to wait for the right relationship than to jump
into a premature marriage.

Fran and Timothy married secretly while they were
in high school. In only a few years the fun and excitement
seemed to disappear, and they finally divorced. Tim was
pretty faithful with support payments for Fran and the
two-year-old she was raising. It wasn't always easy, but she
found a good job and enjoyed an active social life. By the
age of twenty-three, she entered her second marriage with
a new pregnancy well under way.

Cindy was a poor student who looked forward to any
kind of a job as a change from the drudgery of school.
After being a waitress for a while, the ups and downs of
her income convinced her to become a salesperson in a
department store. That wasn't much better. When the
older man she was dating expanded his car lot and suggested getting married and working together, Cindy eagerly
accepted with relief.

Irene lived with Mac for her last two years of college.
There was no question that they would remain together,
but neither was ready to start a family. Nor did they see
the necessity of getting married right after graduation.
They did so several years later, warmly, comfortably, and
with a sense of complete security.

Kayleen earned a master's degree from a top business
school and went right into the ranks of management at a
large aero-space corporation. Soon after that she began
dating one of its executive vice-presidents. Neither of them
was seriously interested in marriage, but after a couple of
years and one episode of a pregnancy neither wanted at
the time, they came to the shocking conclusion that they'd
like to have children and "do the whole thing" after all.

All of these women have something in common.

They were making their own decisions, establishing their unique sexual and lifestyle patterns, and experiencing the changes that would mold much of the rest of their lives. With or without marriage, the possibility of pregnancy was constant for all of them. For every woman in this stage of life it is impossible to second guess in which case a pregnancy will be welcome, and when it will be received as a catastrophe.

The vast majority of young women do not become pregnant from dramatic episodes of promiscuity or rape. They are deeply involved in finding the unique sexual and emotional maturity that will shape the rest of their lives. The effects of pregnancy on their personal growth can be interpreted only by each woman herself. At this stage, more than any other, interpretive formulas cannot and will not work.

Independence, the right to pursue one's own personal goals, and the flexibility to make changes are the keynotes of this stage of life. The likelihood of change adds interest and sometimes problems to the mix. Experimentation is easier, and the freedom to admit mistakes and move in a new direction is greater than at any other time of life. For these reasons, marriage and divorce rates are high at this time, and this age group represents a full 50 percent of the cases seen at the clinic.

Twenty-four to Thirty-four: Active Adulthood and Pursuit of Life's Goals. By the age of twenty-four, most people have chosen their life's goals and begun to work seriously at reaching them. For most men and women, adulthood is a state of self-sufficiency, of being able to provide for oneself and others. Whatever one's goals, whether a family, career, or simply a happy relationship and a good life, reaching for them expands one's senses of reality about what we really can accomplish. This is a period of working to make the right things happen.

Changes in lifestyles, relationships, and residence are not only possible but much in evidence. However, their effects are deeper and frequently more difficult than earlier in life. A ten-year marriage may well contain more reasons for divorce than a two-year one, but without question greater responsibilities are likely to be involved, not the least of which may be several children. Friendships and jobs cultivated over a significant span of time bring their own considerations. The passage of each year brings its own commitments and strengthens previous ones in a woman's thinking about herself and the life she has built. Each major change demands ever increasing care because it may lead to an exchange of problems instead of an elimination of them.

Despite the acceptance of divorce with or without remarriage, despite the fact that a change may be refreshing and necessary, and despite the advantages of mobility and the potential of earning a living elsewhere, in this stage of life women and men begin to become aware of new pitfalls. They start to replace dramatic change with the more deliberate process of modification.

It becomes apparent that all the initial values, benefits, and sources of satisfaction may not have to be discarded altogether. As often as not, the best may be retained and new dimensions built upon them. These may include new jobs, career advancement, or a broader, more gratifying lifestyle. The choice between change or modification becomes a matter of the degree of need to reach in new directions for that elusive quality called contentment.

Denise put it this way: "Don't make me feel guilty. I've gone through a lot of that already, and I still feel it strongly. I've had the two kids I wanted, and then even had a third because my husband wanted a son. Well, that all worked out fine and we're happy. They're in school now. I've done a good job with them and always will. I don't feel free, as such, and don't know that I completely want to be. Things aren't bad, you see, but I have the feeling that I want to enjoy a part of my very own life, and I like it. I want it. More than that, I need it. Starting over with a fourth one, well, it might not drive me completely crazy, but there wouldn't be much left of me . . . for myself, my kids, my husband, or anyone."

The expression of modification rather than dramatic change shows itself in even quieter ways. It may be the product of a lifetime of values built up from within and held dearly. Corrie, for example, was thirty-two. She had been in and out of a one-year marriage in her teens, started working with the telephone company soon after that, and rose to become a supervisor with the prospect of continuing advancement. She was a popular and witty redhead, very much in charge of her life. As far as she was concerned, getting married again for her young son's sake was the silliest thing a woman could do. She liked to date a variety of men and could handle herself in any situation. Then again, she often preferred to spend an evening at home, reading and listening to music. The problem was that most of the men she met were pretty dull. Sometimes she recalled a song that said, "A good man nowadays is hard to find." That always brought a knowing smile to her lips because she had no intention of settling for less.

The one man for whom she might change her life had been married twice and was totally against trying it again. He and Corrie liked each other and enjoyed the time they spent together. Once, though, she slipped with her birth control pills and went through two weeks of panic until her next period was due. Her panic turned out to be justified.

Since she'd already been through it, Corrie was realistic about not trying to force an unwanted marriage out of an unwanted pregnancy. Still, the whole outcome made her very depressed and unhappy. Wouldn't it be easier just to settle down with something halfway decent? On the other hand, she thought seriously about simply having her tubes tied. She went through a really painful evaluation of where her life was going. The whole process was far from easy. "I'm not going to tear it all up now," she finally concluded. "But I'm not ready to quit looking either. Let me go back on the pill. It probably won't matter, but at least for a while I want to keep my options."

Dee, on the other hand, already had a family she loved very much. Some might call her a housewife, but everyone who knew her thought of her as a clever executive in disguise. The effortless, breezy way she ran her household and was always available for her three kids, yet managed to do lots of creative things on her own, was amazing.

"Now look here, Doctor," she said to me, "I don't have a problem with you and I don't want one. You're going to help me, right? We're going to tie my tubes. That's the big contribution I want in my life now. I've thought about it a lot. And Walter? He thinks it's great. He even let me turn in that tacky old wagon for a zippy little sports car. You're not going to tell me I have to have ten kids and be sixty years old, are you? I have three darling children. Love 'em to pieces. But if I get pregnant again I'll just die!"

Most adults have had enough exposure to people, attempted enough relationships, experienced enough failures, and tasted enough success to recognize which of their goals are within reach. Less obvious but of much greater importance is the deeper goal that most of us have: to establish a personal identity that is a reflection of our innermost feelings.

When we recognize this need it is likely to cause life change. It may include the desire for many children, limit their number at successive stages of life, or allow for none at all. Sooner or later it demands attention, and its call tends to become unavoidably clear before the mid-thirties. If and when it signals an additional pregnancy as an intolerable restriction rather than a blessing, then the decision to terminate or permanently prevent this experience becomes more than a matter of careful choice. It becomes an overwhelming command of one's inner needs.

And so, what may seem to be a cold-hearted judgment to take a job, return to school, or wash one's hands of motherhood is very likely the reflection of much stronger forces of identity at work.

Thirty-four–Plus: Consolidation of a Lifestyle. By the early to mid-thirties, the consolidation of a satisfying personal identity has usually replaced the need for a reproductive role that the majority of women have by then felt obligated to play. The most startling feature of what is happening today is that this transition is taking place at younger and younger ages. Only a decade ago, ages forty to forty-five were considered a reasonable time when a woman might gracefully consider giving up her reproductive capacity. Today, this age has moved to the early thirties and it is rapidly dropping into the twenties. By the time a woman has reached thirty-four, in the great majority of cases, she has reevaluated her life and decided to take advantage of the option to expand it by using the newfound freedom that comes when the duties of young motherhood end. No longer does this stage of life demand a graceful fading into the woodwork. Instead, it opens all kinds of new doors.

Not all women or men feel like this. But most women (as well as men) who have not been beaten down by the stress of routine living enjoy this feeling. They still want adventures in life. Their numbers, in both sexes, are increasing.

At the age of thirty-eight, Amanda had no worries about losing her attractiveness. She had a warm and beautiful relationship with her husband, a prominent attorney. They were both involved in many community affairs and were members of an easily recognized list of boards and panels. Their biggest weekly problems were figuring out what social event to fit in where. There was only one painful part of their lives—they had never been able to have children of their own. After several years of trial and failure, they had the good fortune to adopt infant twins, who grew into splendid youngsters and gave them all the joys and headaches any parents can expect.

Mandy and her husband came to the clinic with a mixture of sadness and firm resolve. She had become pregnant after all those years of futility and frustration, and both of them felt that she was in no position to think now of starting the family that had been withheld from her for so long.

After the mid-thirties, a major new lifestyle decision becomes more difficult because the time available to make such an important change decreases with age. The woman or man who contemplates striking out into a different career, changing partners in marriage, or making a definite decision whether to marry or stay single usually considers these options very seriously after this point in life.

At forty-three, Ida was thinking intensely about all of these things. Her sexual life was satisfactory, her husband's interest in her and financial support were fairly good, and she had developed an active life of her own. She had three or four encounters over the years with other men. Physical gratification hadn't been that important, but there had been an amount of extra excitement she couldn't deny. All in all, she felt she had done a really good job in her duties to her husband and family in spite of an occasional adventure. She never allowed her affairs to get out of hand, and she had neither the interest nor the incentive to disrupt her family.

"I feel like an idiot," she said. "After all these years I thought I was falling in love—really in love—a lot different from anything I ever had with my husband. I had nothing to complain about at home, which made it worse. I thought about this man all the time. He wanted me to get a divorce and marry him. I was almost ready to do it until this happened.

"We've known each other for six months," she continued. "He's got problems with his wife. They haven't slept together in years, and now, I've missed *my* period. Anyway, that was a joke I never expected. It turned everything into a nightmare. I feel sick and scared to death."

"What do you want to do?" I asked.

A very long pause made her sigh sound even deeper. "I don't know what I want, exactly. It's more what I don't want. I don't want to let it all go by and disappear. I don't want to say the things I should, like how could I be so stupid, and help me out of this mess so I can go back home and behave forever. I don't want my life to be over and have no more to look forward to than the thrill of social security.

"It must sound worse than it is," she said. "There's more. I don't want to tear up what I've got, not really. And, God help me, no matter how all this works out, I don't want to have a baby. Not now. Not now or ever again. There's a limit to middle-age adolescence. I know. I found it.

"I have too many friends who broke away from their lives. The ones who did it to be free by themselves seem to have done better, all in all. The others who remarried in a month? One seems happy. The rest keep saying something that I simply can't forget. They want to know how it's possible to do the same thing twice—the same man in a different bed, the same nonsense at a different address. It all seemed hardly worth the trip. I'm not any smarter than they are, but I may have learned something even if it did come with a jolt. I'm not sure what it is yet, but there's got to be a better way than this."

Often, such romantic relationships are built on fears of losing youthfulness, with a resulting panic pregnancy. Less dramatic but even more severe are cases in which a woman in her late forties or even early fifties comes to the clinic with a totally unexpected problem.

Edith had fairly regular periods for most of her life. She started skipping two and then three at a time when she turned forty-nine, and then stopped menstruating altogether by the time she was fifty. Both she and her husband had a warm glow about the idea of reaching the time of life when they no longer had to worry about pregnancy but still thoroughly enjoyed their sexual relations. She thought the occasional waves of nausea and irritability were part of the menopause, perhaps a variation of hot flashes. In any event, for peace of mind they seemed a reasonable price. What finally alarmed her enough to visit me in my private practice was the tenderness and swelling of her breasts.

When I told her that her pelvic exam and urinalysis indicated pregnancy, Edith just about went into a state of shock. "I can't be pregnant," she said. "I'm in the menopause. For God's sake, I'm fifty years old. Look at me."

"You know it and I know it. Even your husband knows it," I said, "but this test tells us that you are younger than you thought."

Edith and her husband returned to the office several days later. She was still dazed and her husband didn't know whether to feel proud or silly. "You know," he said, "I had the damndest urge to tell my friends. Then I thought about my children. That wasn't half so bad, but do you know that I have grandchildren? I think any idea of going through with this would be insane. Besides, what about the genetic business? And when *can* we stop worrying about pregnancy?"

"There is an increase in genetic problems after forty," I said. "And menopause does not mean that you can't get pregnant. The only rule of thumb is to be careful about contraception for a full two years after periods seem to have quit."

"How often does this happen?" was his last question.

"Often enough to be careful," was the only realistic answer.

Personal Needs Are the Common Denominator. It is easy and sometimes helpful to think about pregnancy in terms of age groupings, degrees of maturity, marital status, changing personal goals, and the like. But the helpfulness of generalities stops short of helping any individual.

Most women can become pregnant at any time during an average forty years of fertility. What might that great interval imply? That every woman should have forty children? That hardly seems reasonable.

The most sensible approach is that women need the benefit of the broadest possible range of options for motherhood. Why? Bringing one child or many into the world should be done in as close to ideal circumstances as possible, in the best interests of everyone involved. The best conditions are likely to occur for different women at different times in their lives. To many, it may occur often. To others, not at all. Judgments on these matters may or may not be made from a woman's thoughts alone. In this day and time, her needs must be valued first.

Unfortunately, those forty years offer ample opportunities for pregnancy to occur in less than ideal, and often frankly adverse, conditions. For too many years, before legalization, the outcome of this kind of tragedy was destined to be further suffering, injury, or death.

Today, there is help. Today, there has emerged compassion for a woman as she exists, with recognition and respect for her needs. Today, those forty years can truly be thought of as options, rather than threats. When chance and circumstance cast pregnancy as a misfortune, there are professionals to whom a woman may openly turn with faith and trust.

II

MEDICAL AND EMOTIONAL UNDERSTANDING

3

DISCOVERING THE PREGNANCY

Recognition of Pregnancy

From the first minute Martha suspected she might be pregnant, she began a total review of her place in the world and her ability to bring another child into it. She was twenty-nine, in good health, and her family was happy and relatively well off. She had two children and a husband who cared about all of them. She couldn't help but feel insecurities, doubts, and anxieties about going through another pregnancy.

The fact that there were no major problems in having her first two children was encouraging, but each pregnancy was a new adventure. Deep inside she somehow knew that this pregnancy was welcome—very welcome. But she decided that she still needed the reassurance of her husband because a new place of importance would have to be made alongside their other two children. His reaction was, "Oh, my God! I'm not sure how, but we'll work everything out."

Whether a woman faces the prospect of pregnancy for the first or fifth time, its impact on her life is very great. That impact may be pleasant if the woman's circumstances permit her to accept it with happiness. It may be tolerated and accepted if she lives under some stress and uncertainty. Or, she might not be able to accept it if her life is difficult. Whatever the decision, no woman takes lightly the immediate impact and the long-range responsibility of bringing a child into the world.

Motherhood Desires and Inner Conflicts. Sarah did not have the luxury of a husband who was present. This steady, responsible woman in her late twenties provided the emotional and financial sustenance for her children by herself. Her only help was the hit-or-miss child-support checks from her ex-husband. It was bad enough that they were more miss than hit. The fact that she had no one to give her the deep emotional support she herself needed was much worse. These needs were filled to a slight degree by a man she knew whom she would never marry. She was not a swinger, but needed the comfort of a warm relationship.

One day, the suspicion that she was pregnant converted a bright aspect of her existence into the possibility of a catastrophe. Sarah loved her children very much. She did not want to think about having an abortion. But she knew that she was quite alone, and could not visualize any way that she could keep the pregnancy, if it were true.

Sarah shut her mind and rejected her suspicions. She didn't even take her first missed period seriously until she missed the second one. She had one episode of heavy bleeding during this time, and several traces of spotting. Each one made her hope that her period might have been delayed, or that she was going through this suspenseful torture as a lesson in being more careful. Then, when she couldn't deny it any longer, it took her three more weeks to summon the courage to make an appointment to confirm her pregnancy.

A positive pregnancy test and pelvic exam fixed her pregnancy at eleven weeks' gestation. Sarah's reaction was the totally silent tears of one who is condemned. "My children," she finally said as she lay there. "I can't let this happen to my children."

Sarah managed to face her situation after a great deal of inner turmoil. "I looked at it in every direction," she said, "and this is the only thing I can do. I have two children I must raise now and no husband to help me. I can't do it any other way."

The trite phrase, maternal instinct, does not explain this woman's strong feelings. Sarah was very unhappy after the procedure and cried for the child that might have been. She took comfort in the realization that she would not be crying if she had used contraceptives to prevent her pregnancy. She felt much more comfort from her concern for her existing children. Ultimately, she left the clinic with the understanding that the two children she already had at home needed her more.

Sarah's dilemma paralleled that of so many women who must face an abortion. The children who are already there may be already receiving all the strength, resources, and support a woman can give. Keeping a pregnancy may hurt rather than help an entire family. In this case, a mother must choose wisely and in light of the unique problems that exist in her life.

Denying an Unwanted Pregnancy: A Frequent Problem.
Sarah came within a week of compounding her problems enormously. She almost fell into the trap that waits for women who reject the first sign of an unexpected pregnancy, *missing a period or having an abnormal period.*

As Sarah explained it: "I don't want to be pregnant ... not like this ... I was so afraid I didn't want to know what was happening." She knew the truth of the stories that worrying about being pregnant or even having an upset daily routine can lead to irregular or missed periods. She also knew that swollen breasts and some nausea (morning or otherwise) can go along with pregnancy, but can also be caused by any disruption of menstruation.

Because of her fears, Sarah didn't want to face reality, and she almost delayed confirming her pregnancy beyond the critical point of twelve weeks. Women who are like her—who go through a prolonged denial or inner struggle over what to do—often wind up needing a second-trimester procedure. This is a serious mistake. After twelve weeks, pregnancy termination becomes a hospital procedure. It is more involved medically, more expensive financially, and more traumatic emotionally.

A woman who delays discovering or dealing with her pregnancy until the second trimester can least afford the extra difficulties that result. The twenty-seven hospitals in my area perform virtually no second-trimester procedures. This situation is much the same all over the country. A woman in the second trimester must often travel hundreds of miles to find a hospital in which she will be helped.

If a woman is in the least concerned about whether she might be pregnant, she should confirm or rule out pregnancy as rapidly as possible. This will give her time to arrive at her best decision, if she is pregnant, without being pushed into the medical system's problems in providing a second-trimester procedure.

All Bleeding Is Not Menstruation. Edelle hadn't missed a period, but her breasts were swollen and she was sick from nausea in the mornings. Her doctor wanted to wait and see if she missed her next period, but she called us and scheduled a pregnancy test. It was positive, and she was stunned to learn, from her pelvic exam, that she was twelve weeks pregnant. "How can I be this far along and never miss a period?" she asked.

There are many causes of vaginal bleeding other than menstruation. Bleeding may occur because of irritation or infection of the vagina, cervix, or uterus. It may be caused by an irregularity in a woman's menstrual clock, when she deviates from the exact hormonal sequence required to release an egg from an ovary. It can occur because of a reason like transient stress, or as is often the case, for no specific reason at all.

Menstrual bleeding itself results from the lining of the uterus being built up in a cycle every month, then being sloughed off when the implantation of a pregnancy does not occur. I've heard that explanation answered a thousand times by patients who say: "You mean that all this mess is because I am set up to become pregnant every month?" Contrary to our thinking about the role of women in today's world, the answer is yes.

The most important bleeding that might be confused with menstrual bleeding occurs in the early stages of pregnancy. Most often, it results from the process of the egg's implantation into the same lining of the uterus about which we just spoke. The amount of bleeding may be light staining, it may be as much as a normal period, or it may be quite a bit heavier.

Most physicians recognize this fact and would so instruct their patients in response to a question in a written examination. In practice, however, the failure to inform women about this bleeding is of overwhelming importance in causing a great many second-trimester problems. One out of three women have a variable amount of bleeding at or shortly after the time of implantation. This is the most significant cause of women's underestimating the suspected length of their pregnancy.

The net results of this phenomenon are devastating

in terms of impact as well as numbers affected. Every day women appear at the clinic with clearly marked calendars proving that they must be seven weeks along rather than eleven. A truly great tragedy is in store for the woman who must have her pregnancy terminated and thinks she is at ten weeks but turns out to be at fourteen weeks. The problems she faces in the sudden change from the first trimester to the second are enormous.

It is impossible to offer a fail-safe formula for evaluating this kind of bleeding. The best advice is that any suspicion of pregnancy and any abnormal period should be checked with a physician as soon as possible. No woman in this position should wait for her next period.

Of course, it is more convenient for a busy doctor to save a woman an office visit and tell her in a quick phone call: "Check with me in a month if you miss another period." It's more convenient for a woman to agree with this, and defer a showdown with reality. And it's more convenient for both patient and doctor to rely on a calendar and a haphazard pregnancy test without confirming it by a pelvic examination. However, these "conveniences" often result in a situation where many women learn about their pregnancies long after the point where a difficult decision becomes severe.

How Many Weeks Pregnant?

There has been a lot of discussion about the weeks of pregnancy being very important for a woman to know. To a woman who has to regard a pregnancy as a major threat to the stability of her life, this knowledge is more than just helpful, it is critical.

The First-trimester Crisis. Penny was upset at herself for forgetting to take her birth control pills for several days at a time. She knew the symptoms well from four previous pregnancies. These were wonderful additions to her life, but her youngest child had finally reached kindergarten and she didn't want to start over at the age of thirty-three. Besides, four children was all she and her husband could afford. It wasn't that a fifth child would strain their budget. It was already stretched. Another major expense would completely destroy it.

Her obstetrician, a pleasant but elderly fellow, had no idea of the circumstances of her life. Penny wanted to keep it that way, but knew that his determination of the length of her pregnancy was extremely important.

"Good to see you again," he said. "The way you keep coming back I'll never make any money treating you for infertility."

"Lord, do I know," she muttered quietly between her teeth. "I need to find out exactly how far along I am," she said out loud.

"Lose your calendar?" he asked. "Probably too busy taking care of your family."

"Please get on with it," she muttered again to herself. As soon as the exam was over she asked, "How far along am I?"

"Oh, I don't know. Between eight and ten or eleven weeks. What difference does it make? Nobody delivers when they're due, except by accident. All you need to know is the right month so you don't take a vacation."

Penny knew that it would be a waste of time trying to pin down anything more. She had sense enough to make an immediate seventy-mile trip to the nearest up-to-date clinic to get an accurate answer.

Until the recent advent of legal abortion, it was not worth training gynecologists how to tell the subtle differences in the size of the uterus between eight and nine weeks, ten or eleven weeks, or, most important, between twelve and thirteen weeks. Even today, only a moderate number of gynecologists and a much smaller number of general practitioners have developed the skill of sizing an early pregnancy accurately. This statement is not a criticism. This is a very specialized skill. Most doctors have had little use for this information in the past.

Women also need to know that the number of weeks they are told is measured *from the first day of their last normal menstrual period*. Tarra, for example, began menstrual bleeding on the first day of August and was found to be pregnant on the fifteenth of September. She was told that she was six weeks pregnant. In actuality, conception probably occurred around the fifteenth of August.

This method of dating a pregnancy may not seem accurate, but it has a good rationale. First, the uterus begins preparing for pregnancy from the onset of menstruation. By the time the conception occurs the uterus is already two weeks prepared to receive the newly fertilized egg. Second, it is impossible to date pregnancy from the moment of ovulation because there isn't any way to know when a woman ovulated in any particular menstrual cycle. Finally, trying to guess which of many occasions of intercourse produced the pregnancy may reveal some fascinating sexual histories, but they have little medical value. As a result, the size of the uterus from the last menstrual period is used to determine the number of weeks of gestation.

In its main impact this means that a woman has, on average, two weeks less than she thinks before the first trimester ends. As soon as she misses her third period she has entered the second trimester.

Hopefully, one day all women will know that they need to have the number of weeks of pregnancy determined as soon as they suspect they have an unwanted pregnancy. The time between this suspicion and the end of the first trimester is often very short. Women who don't do this risk turning the crisis of an unwanted pregnancy into a major personal emergency. They are playing with a fire that will almost certainly burn them badly.

The Second-trimester Emergency. Yvonne was raped in a secluded part of her college campus. The emotional upheaval that followed proved almost more than she could handle. She dropped out of classes for two weeks just to regain her composure. Missing a period or two after all the turmoil didn't seem unusual to her or her friends who knew what she was going through. With the best of intentions they tried to reassure her that in all probability nothing was seriously wrong. She was terrified that a pregnancy was bound to add to her problems, but couldn't face this possibility enough to get a pregnancy test.

After missing her third period she finally made an appointment at the clinic. The words "fourteen weeks" fell on her head like a hammer. It took several minutes before "We will have to refer you someplace else" got through to her. Panic tumbled over understanding like a wave exploding on a rocky shore.

"Don't refer me," she pleaded. "Help me now. It wasn't my fault. I trust you. I'll sign anything. Please, please help me."

It took a few minutes for Yvonne to settle down. She wiped her eyes and tossed her head, whisking her long blond hair away from her face. I wanted to say something positive and comforting, but my next words hit that pretty head like another hammer blow.

"Six to nine hundred dollars! And a hospital two hundred miles away! That's impossible! I can't borrow that, except from my parents, and they still don't know anything about what's happened to me—and I don't want them to. What am I going to do?" The second wave had hit.

By the time it subsided there was only one more to go. Yvonne's suddenly calm voice reflected the numbness all this distressing information was causing. "Why do I have to wait another month?"

"Because the procedure is safer and more effective at eighteen than at fourteen weeks."

"That's the end of the road," she said slowly. She bit her lip and her look of determination grew until her expression called loudly for the last bit of advice.

"Don't do it, Yvonne. You'll only add to your problems. It will hurt your parents a lot more to get word that you're hemorrhaging in the middle of the night in an emergency room, and it will hurt you to wind up with an infection that can mess up your chances of having a baby when you really want one."

Her head snapped around. "How did you know—?"

"I've been there," I said.

"But why do I have to travel two hundred miles to get this procedure done? We have perfectly fine hospitals here, don't we?"

"Yes, our hospitals are fine, but they are basically very much against anything to do with abortion. The personnel frequently reflect these attitudes. As far as I'm concerned, going there would be a terrible mistake. I've seen too many patients hurt by careless, prejudiced remarks."

I shrugged my shoulders helplessly. "I have to insist that you arrange to travel to a hospital that will do it right, because that is the only way to get the kind of treatment that will help you more than hurt."

In the second trimester the cost of a procedure may

immediately triple, at the very least. Instead of a five-minute procedure, the average duration jumps to nineteen hours. The commonly used technique is instillation of medication into the uterus halfway through the second trimester, followed by many hours of waiting that climax in a miniature labor.

It is my considered and firm opinion that this must be performed in a hospital or specifically approved facility, not just because of the law but because of medical safety. Mortality rates triple entering the second trimester, even under ideal circumstances.

Despite public statements of no prohibition against abortion, the greatest majority of hospitals are unwilling to provide this service at all. With some justification, this situation has been referred to as a quiet conspiracy. In the formal structure of many hospitals, determined anti-abortionists have succeeded in intimidating the institution by threats of bad publicity, picketing, physician resistance, and other nonsense. I have spoken to quite a few hospital administrators who would be more than happy to expend their efforts in properly caring for second-trimester cases, even if this meant caring for them separately in a presently unused ward or wing. These administrators have beds to spare and financial problems to solve, but the opposition of a few vociferous staff or board members is enough to kill the idea. Good-intentioned or not, administrators cannot sustain a fight on this issue. They have to get along, if for no other reason than to preserve their jobs. In the press of principle versus practicality, the path of least resistance has proved stronger than an unmet patient need.

The majority of the scattered hospitals that permit second-trimester procedures do not have specially trained personnel to assist the patient. In first-trimester clinics we have found a wide variety of emotional needs in women at this time and have tailored our care, personnel, and policies to meet them. In a hospital, where a woman in the second trimester has needs equal to or greater than a woman in the first trimester, personnel generally do not understand the emotional needs that accompany an abortion.

On occasion, women delay checking for a pregnancy because they assume they are in the menopause. "I don't believe this!" Chris said. At forty-six, she was married, the mother of two children, and the regional manager of nearly two dozen department stores for a national corporation. "I thought that I quit having periods because I was too old," she said in shock. "My mother went into the menopause at forty-six so I thought that I would too. There's just no way I can keep this pregnancy."

There isn't any valid familial clock for menopause. This is another misconception that can cause delays and escalate a first-trimester crisis into a second-trimester emergency. By the time she discovered her pregnancy, Chris was beyond the first trimester.

Confirming the Pregnancy and Consulting a Doctor. Every pregnancy should be confirmed or ruled out as soon as it is suspected, whether the intention is to keep it or terminate it. Exactly what does that mean? It is much more than a phone call and a pregnancy test. It should include a pelvic exam by a doctor to determine the duration of the pregnancy and provide sound medical advice in the event of physical problems.

If the pregnancy is to be continued, that information may be valuable for prescribing medication, ending the use of birth control pills, determining what to do if an IUD is in place, testing for blood types, or other necessary actions. A variety of tests, diagnoses, and treatment may be advisable for either the mother or the pregnancy, to give her and her child the best health and the best delivery.

If a pregnancy cannot be continued, the length of gestation is a major factor in the impact the pregnancy has on the woman. Gestation is determined only by a pelvic exam. If this confirmation is delayed for too long, it may determine a woman's ultimate decision. One chubby thirteen-year-old was brought in by her mother, who noticed she was gaining weight and wearing looser fitting clothes. This teenager's pregnancy test was positive, but her pelvic exam was startling. She was a full eight months pregnant and delivered in a matter of weeks. I have seen this repeated a frightening number of times, mostly in young teenage women. It is as big a shock to a teenager's family as it is to her.

Confirmation of a pregnancy is easily available. Most health departments and abortion clinics offer pregnancy tests free or at minimal fees, while private physicians charge normal fees. The old days of testing with rabbits and frogs are gone. A two-minute, relatively efficient chemical test is used. This test reacts to the presence of a hormone called CGH.

The effects of this quick exercise in the lab are too far reaching for it to be done improperly. The most common reason for a negative test that should have been positive is a urine sample diluted by too much liquid consumed by a woman. This is why the test is usually done with an early-morning specimen.

No lab technician or nurse should ever guess at the results of a pregnancy test. If there is any question in reading a test and the diagnosis is, "Maybe she's pregnant and maybe she's not," the patient should be asked to return for retesting. No patient should ever be annoyed at hearing that news.

A pregnancy test should not be given alone, because a concurring pelvic exam is absolutely essential. A negative test is not always reliable and should be checked by direct examination. If the test is positive, there are several conditions that may be present other than a routine, normal pregnancy. These include dangerous conditions that may harm a woman's health, such as ectopic pregnancies, which occur in abnormal locations, such as in a tube or in the abdominal cavity. There are certain tumors that arise from pregnancy, such as hydatid moles, choreocarcinomas, and teratomas. Although these are rare, any of them can lead to serious problems and even death. It is the pelvic exam that leads a doctor to diagnose an abnormality or assure a woman that she can expect a normal pregnancy. A woman's health and medical needs can be evaluated only by a physician's direct observation.

About 5 to 10 percent of all normal pregnancies end in miscarriages, which doctors call spontaneous abortions. I've said that just as all bleeding does not indicate a period, so all bleeding in pregnancy does not indicate a miscarriage. I have cared for women through pregnancy who literally had bath towels full of blood. These women had perfectly normal deliveries with perfectly normal children. Other women have lost pregnancies spontaneously with no more than a few spots of blood as an indication. The woman who feels that she must have a pregnancy terminated and who is also bleeding should never try undue waiting in the hopes that the pregnancy will terminate itself.

Who Else Should You Involve?

All the doctor said was: "Congratulations, you're pregnant." Marie was stunned and almost fainted. For a moment she wasn't sure what she felt.

The problem of an unexpected pregnancy is different for every woman who encounters it. Some women can easily decide what to do. For other women, this problem threatens to shake the foundations of their world. Their emotional stability weakens because they react more intensely to the pressure of finding an answer.

It is comforting to reach out for help with this decision, if the right kind of help is available. Other people bring perspective to the situation, the ability to help without becoming clouded by emotions, stress, or pressures. Such objectivity often makes it easier to help other people than to solve our own problems.

A brilliant scientist may be able to solve complex equations, but need suggestions on even the smallest personal decisions, such as what shirt to wear on a particular day. If a woman with an unexpected pregnancy is lucky, she may need no more than a friend with whom she can talk out her situation and hear her own words expressing her feelings. This way some fortunate women discover that they already know what is good and right for themselves. The reassurance from the people around them that, indeed, they know what they should do confirms their judgment. Such reassurance is important, because it can help us live with our decisions.

When a woman's reassurance comes from within herself, it certainly simplifies her situation. If it comes from a professional who helps her think her situation through, such as a physician, psychiatrist, minister, or social worker, it serves the same purpose and is of great value.

The basic criteria in deciding who to involve are not complicated. One question must be answered. Will those persons place *your* needs above their own? If they cannot do this, if their needs come first, it may be a mistake to approach them. Involving someone who will attempt to make your decision for you, or subtly inviting someone to do this out of a reluctance to decide for yourself, is no shortcut to the best decision.

Valerie ran and owned half a chain of women's clothing shops. She loved her husband and felt very close to him. Despite the fact that much of the excitement of the early parts of their marriage had mellowed into an easygoing sense of comfort she was never in the least bit interested in looking for an affair or even an adventure. On one unexpected occasion she found herself overcome by a rush of excitement that she hadn't felt in many years. She regretted the incident and made up her mind that she would never discuss it, but would suffer the feelings of her own guilt in silence. When she learned that she was pregnant this thought became an impossibility.

When I saw Valerie she needed quite a bit more advice than the average woman with an unwanted pregnancy. After learning that she was pregnant she had turned to her business associate as a friend, never dreaming that the information would be used to blackmail her into selling out her half-ownership in the business. Valerie had refused at first, but after her partner started dropping hints to her husband that Valerie was having an ongoing affair with several men, she gave in and sold out.

This story may sound extreme, but it is a clear example of whom *not* to confide in: someone who puts her own needs first.

At the other extreme is the woman who won't tell anyone. Cheryl's divorce had been a desperate escape from a horrible marriage. Her husband used to beat her, and even after their divorce he continued to harass her with phone calls and threats. With her parents' help, she got a court injunction that kept him from bothering her. After that, her life returned to normal. She liked the first man she went out with, and they made love on their third date. She used no contraceptive because she hadn't planned on sexual relations that quickly.

When I first met Cheryl she was in a state of agitation, though she hadn't missed even one period.

"I know coming here so soon must look stupid," she said, "but you have no idea how upset I am. This is the first time in two years I liked anybody, and I can't stand the possibility that I might be pregnant now. Is there some way you could make sure I'm not pregnant, even though it's this early?"

We talked about the "morning-after pill." I explained that it may make a woman feel sick, is certainly not foolproof, and if it is to be of value it has to be used within twenty-four hours after intercourse. We talked a bit about menstrual extraction (also known as menstrual regulation) procedures, which are miniature D & Cs. I explained that these procedures involve just about as much as a regular abortion in the first trimester, and that their efficiency rate is highly questionable. If, in point of fact, she was pregnant, the whole thing might have to be done again.

During this discussion Cheryl became relieved that she could talk about her overall problems freely. Her biggest concern was that she felt horribly low and alone. We discussed these feelings at length.

"Have you talked about this with anyone else?" I asked.

"No, I can't. I don't want to talk to my parents. They've been too nice already and they don't need more aggravation from me."

"How about your boyfriend?"

"I don't want him to know either. It wasn't his fault. He didn't mean to do anything to get me upset, and he's got his own problems. He's divorced too, and he's taking care of his little girl. Anyway, I don't want his attention because I'm pregnant. If he likes me, I don't want this to be the reason for it."

"Would you tell him if you were sure you are pregnant? Or do you want to discuss it with anyone else?"

"No . . . it's no one else's problem. It's my problem. It seems that any time I get close to people I get hurt. If I ever marry again, I don't want to think that a pregnancy had anything to do with it."

Cheryl was determined to deal with her own problems in her own way. She was pregnant and did have an abortion after all. She handled herself well but the whole episode was more difficult than it might have been because she kept everything to herself.

The majority of women of all ages are close to trustworthy people who care about them. Teresa was one of these lucky ones. The people surrounding her really helped. She was only seventeen and became pregnant just before finishing high school. She had the luxury of a concerned boyfriend who didn't want to see her hurt. He came with her to tell her parents. Although this was far from a comfortable experience, her parents did not condemn her as a horrible child with no sense at all. In fact, they said that they felt guilty about her situation, too. They knew that she was deeply involved and that the most she was able to do was hint of her need for birth control. If they had been quicker to realize the potential of pregnancy, and hadn't put out of their minds the possibility of this happening to their daughter, they might have prevented the whole situation.

Her parents came with Teresa and her boyfriend to the clinic. There we confirmed that she was pregnant and counseled all these people as to her various alternatives. The results of this decision were satisfactory because everyone cared and supported Teresa in what she thought was best.

Those who would tend to judge or simply hurt the pregnant woman should be excluded and not even told of the situation. It is none of their business. The people who really can help are those who want to contribute to the quality of the woman's life rather than to force her to follow their own views and needs. The woman who wants to carry this burden alone, with no more than the help of the professionals she consults, has every right to her decision as well.

One additional guideline is important. If the father of the pregnancy is involved in an ongoing relationship with the woman, as is the case most of the time, then he usually should be included in the decision. Answering the questions "How will I feel about this person and how will he feel about me a year from now?" and "How will this decision affect our individual lives?" helps evaluate his response in advance. If it is likely that those answers are not positive or that his response may be hurtful, then including him is more questionable.

The use of these guidelines is intensely personal. The question of whom to involve in this situation will not fit a formula. The reach for help can be exploratory, if necessary. The best people to turn to are those who will express the most objective concern and wisdom.

Securing the Help Needed. Asking for help of any kind is hard for many people. Asking for it from parents, a husband, or a boyfriend poses an extra problem: Their help may be limited because they are emotionally involved. Does that mean they may not want to help? No. Does it mean that they are more likely to make the problem worse? No. It means that they will need to express their own feelings, perhaps in simple words, perhaps at great length. This reaction is understandable and should be expected.

Most women feel that their parents, husbands, or boyfriends want the best for them. Yet they usually hesitate before revealing an unexpected pregnancy. They may be afraid of losing the love or respect of these people. They tend to carry a sense of guilt, deserved or not, for having let down someone important to them. This may be unfair, illogical, and painful, but it is a reaction that definitely does exist.

If a woman wants to be realistic, she should expect the opposite: *Parents, husbands, or boyfriends are most likely to want the same thing that the pregnant woman wants,* whether it is keeping or ending the pregnancy. They are most likely to feel that way for exactly the same reasons the woman does. That statement is not a rationalization to make a pregnant woman feel better. It is true.

A woman's first step in going to those most intimately concerned should be her own evaluation of what would be best for her. Once that understanding is figured out, whether alone or with the help of friends or professionals, then a judgment on the merits of confiding can be made reasonably. When this is done it is more than an appeal for support. It is a test of the strengths or weaknesses of the relationship, and it may influence its future or even its survival. Simply put, if a woman feels that the hope and desire is there, she may open her heart freely. If she feels that there is little or no hope for help from the relationship, she would do best to look for support elsewhere.

Those who care will respond well. Those who do not may show just that. The fear of finding out how things really are in a relationship is a valid reason for hesitating, but positive support is what most women discover. Parents, a husband, or a boyfriend are not likely to oppose abortion of an unwanted pregnancy if that is a woman's choice.

A test for deep relationships may not be easy because the results may not be close to the heart's desire. More often than not, they will be. When the chance of help and sincere interest appears to be greater than the chance of rejection and all that it implies, then this appeal should be made honestly and without fear.

The Choices Before You

The most difficult moment of many unexpected pregnancies is when the people involved realize that there are only three choices in this situation: keeping the baby; having it and putting it up for adoption; or terminating the pregnancy. "Isn't there something else?" is a question we are asked many times a week. The answer is, "No."

But what can help? Our answer is alternative counseling, which reviews all the reasons for and against every one of these three choices. These counseling sessions sometimes last for several hours and often include the husband or boyfriend, parents, and occasionally, a friend. The counselors go into depth, into feelings about the pregnancy, the woman's relationships, what situation she wants in life, her desires for the future, and the complete picture of what that pregnancy means to her. This is a serious and significant moment for every woman who encounters it, because she is really deciding where her life is going.

This decision is not easy and tears are common. Few people possess absolute certainty and total wisdom. There is almost always some room for doubt, and these doubts can break out to the surface in reflections of what might have been if our world were a better place.

Counseling is important because it keeps the strong points and the weak points of the decision in perspective. That perspective, based on the real certainty that a woman carefully considered all of her alternatives, is a source of valuable reassurance for many years to come. If this decision is made thoughtfully, with concern for all the feelings and people involved, a woman can look back on it and feel that it was the best she could do. No person can expect more than that.

This kind of decision is a turning point and a source of strength for many women. It can sum up who a woman is, what she wants in life, where she is going, the kinds of relationships that are meaningful to her. Everything she has been and has the potential to become enters this equation. Its outcome is a reflection of a woman's deepest desires in her life.

Keeping a Pregnancy. Keeping a pregnancy and bringing a baby into the world can offer gratifications equaled by few other experiences. More often than ever before, a woman's choice is not difficult because the majority of pregnancies today are welcome and happy events. The availability of contraception to many women over the last generation has begun to make pregnancy largely a wanted event for the first time in history. We have not fully developed or put birth control into universal availability, however. Until we reach such an enlightened day, a question mark still arises when a pregnancy is unexpected and conflicts with the realities that a woman faces in her day-to-day life.

Every woman is unique and decides in her own way. A woman who is single and supporting herself or divorced and the sole provider for her children may decide to keep a pregnancy. A woman with children, a stable marriage, and adequate financial resources may decide to terminate a pregnancy. Individual decisions do not fit formulas. The balance a woman feels is best for her and the other people in her world, her desire to keep the pregnancy, and the kind of life she would like to live in the future make up her ultimate reality.

It may seem like heresy for a woman to consider

why she should keep her pregnancy. Nothing could be further from the truth. What can and should be accomplished is a personal evaluation that leads to a stronger and more certain decision by a woman herself, that in light of all her choices and feelings, she is making the right decision for her life.

There are sound medical and emotional benefits that a considered decision might provide. The woman who wants to keep her pregnancy can face it better both immediately and over the many years to come if she has evaluated herself, her feelings, and the feelings of the people in her life. A decision of this sort may help her to eliminate problems, nagging anxieties, and strengthen the positive relationships in her life long before the actual birth of her child occurs.

From the moment most pregnancies are discovered, there are seven to eight months of gestation until the baby is born. That time can be used very effectively for thinking, planning, talking, and in general preparing for the addition of a new life to a woman's family. This time and these efforts can have much greater value than the business of attending an occasional parents' class and knitting little things.

Emotionally secure decisions help everyone. The phenomenon of postpartum depression—the feeling of loss, sadness, or anxiety that sometimes occurs after a baby is born—is still being studied. It may well prove to be the result of inadequate self-evaluation concerning a pregnancy and how it relates to a woman's life. Since legal abortion the phenomenon of postabortal depression has been studied for the first time. Amazingly, it reveals much less guilt, depression, and negative reactions from having an abortion than from giving birth to a baby. This is obviously contrary to what many would expect. But a simple explanation does exist: The woman who has an abortion must seriously consider her decision first. The fact that she has to think these things through will usually give her an exceedingly strong pillar of self-understanding that protects her from many anxieties and questions in the future. If this need for thoughtfulness exists in terminating a pregnancy, the decision to maintain a pregnancy certainly deserves no less.

Adoption. The choice between adoption and abortion is likely to be made under pressure, both internal and from other people, and the alternative that is chosen can affect a woman for the rest of her life.

Either decision may produce the feeling that a woman has done her very best under the circumstances and can live with her decision, or it may produce years of doubt, self-torture, and recrimination. How a woman will feel depends on the adequacy of the counseling available to her. Thoroughness in exploring every avenue makes the difference between whether a woman can live with her decision or may suffer from it later.

Many women choose adoption over abortion because it seems to be a "nicer" choice. In a way it seems more wholesome, though certainly more difficult in terms of time, absence, exposure to an uncomfortable role, and demonstration of a problem to the world. It is the more socially acceptable choice to a few people who have not had to go through carrying a pregnancy and giving birth to a child, only to give it away. That decision may carry even greater repercussions than abortion, because living with adoption amounts to living with a lot of haunting questions in one's mind, questions that can pursue one for years.

These are not comfortable thoughts. They often are the parts of this decision that are suppressed or overlooked. But since these problems do exist, there is an answer.

High-quality adoption agencies have professional counselors who, with warmth and confidence, help each woman
face her unique concerns. Most adoption agencies offer
this kind of care because they are concerned about the
emotional welfare of the mother years after the actions of
the moment are completed.

Reputable agencies make careful studies to evaluate
prospective parents. This is tedious and time-consuming,
but when it is lacking every party involved with an adoption must be very, very guarded. Any indication of hesi-
tancy to demonstrate proficiency in caring for the newborn,
in helping the pregnant woman make a thorough review of her decision, or in total and absolute secrecy of
the identity of both the natural mother and the adopting
parents must be viewed as possible evidence of nonpro-
fessional activity and should be carefully checked out. On
the other hand, agencies that do all this have put the
patient first and deserve the credit and respect of the
community.

Some agencies, unfortunately, put their own interests
first. Their primary goals are quick transactions with a
minimum of social or emotional involvement. These
agencies should be avoided, if possible. So should those
dealing with unborns or newborns for exorbitant fees,
despite superficial niceties like matching hair color and
eye color. This statement is not a blanket condemnation
of expensive adoption services, but it is a strong word of
caution.

A word should also be said about the harm that can
come from informal adoption of the offspring of friends or
relatives with all parties knowing each other. This is likely
to lead to emotional upset to all the adults, and worst of
all, can cause unlimited turmoil for the growing child.

The choice of adoption is easily available for women
who want it. There are long waiting lists of couples who

desperately want to care for and raise a child. It is one of today's facts of life that not many children are available for adoption. Contraception has prevented many unwanted pregnancies. The legalization of abortion has given women a reprieve from unwanted motherhood. But some women are not good candidates for abortion. These are often young women who say they will feel guilty for the rest of their lives and sometimes there are deep emotional reasons.

Billie Jo was one of these women. She came to the clinic for a pregnancy test and the chance to talk it all over. Our counselors came to the conclusion that this young woman had equated the agony of having and losing a child with some form of punishment for having fallen in love with the wrong person. She was not emotionally unbalanced. The programing and conditioning of her life left her little choice. She paid the penitence of her decision at a secluded home for unwed mothers.

Billie Jo's attitude turned her problem pregnancy into a minor catastrophe, and her needs for punishment forced a routine delivery to become a psychiatric nightmare. Her emotional recovery left her in a shambles. She had a need for those shambles because the pain of it all made her feel like a better person. There were other young women at the home who didn't seem to be that upset and even enjoyed themselves from time to time. She couldn't understand them, and felt like she was doing the right thing.

Abortion: The Last Resort. When keeping a pregnancy and adoption have been considered carefully and are unacceptable or unrealistic, then abortion is an acceptable last resort. If a woman cannot keep a pregnancy and reaches this last possible choice, an abortion becomes nothing less than the best way available for her to maintain the quality and dignity of her life.

No matter what a woman's age, bringing a baby into the world is a serious responsibility for all concerned. It can be a painful experience, if a woman and her family are unprepared, to have a baby suddenly dependent on them for all its needs for many years.

The young teenager who has the attitude that pregnancy is wonderful is seen frequently in the clinic. She might want to keep her pregnancy because, she feels, having a child will make her an "instant" adult." She won't have to listen to her mommy because she will be a mommy all by herself. This attitude may be fantasy but occurs often. It is a good example of an immature woman making a decision without considering the responsibilities that go along with it.

Another question of personal responsibility is found in, "What am I doing to the children I already have?" Some people condemn a woman with three children and an irresponsible husband, living on a minimum income, for not wanting to bring a fourth child into the world. The events of pregnancy, childbirth, and child rearing have powerful effects on a couple's relationship, and may push a marriage too far. Then the whole family is the loser.

The bottom line of this decision is usually based on what is best for the quality of a woman's or a family's life, rather than its quantity. The judgment of what produces the best quality must be reserved for those who are intimately involved. *No one else has a right to make that judgment, because no one else has to live with its results.*

4

LET ME HELP YOU THROUGH YOUR CRISIS

The Emotional Strain of Making a Decision

"I really love children, and if things were better, I'd like to have this one. But this is so involved. It is so terribly impossible. Going through with it wouldn't be fair to me or anyone else."

These are phrases heard constantly at the clinic, with a wide range of personal problems filling in the blanks. Some of the stories are very complex, like Bonnie's. In her late teens she had to be put into an institution, where she was raped by an attendant obviously sicker than she. Then there's Tang Hue's story. She found that the material side of living in the United States was better than conditions in Vietnam. Her children were accepted as Americans but she was not. Once her husband was back in this country, the big-breasted appeal of American women recaptured his interest. She had become the world's loneliest baby machine and simply wanted to go home. Most stories are much more simple, but equally deep to the women involved. Quite often, the simpler the story, the more difficult may be the decision.

One factor makes many decisions about problem pregnancies very difficult. There does exist the strong and constantly reinforced feeling that all women are supposed to have children and that that is always supposed to be a joyous event. This formula works fine when it fits the lives of particular women, couples, or families. But it breaks down in confusion, then disruption, then chaos, when twisted and bent to fit all women at all times.

A related problem is the idea that every pregnancy is gratifying to every woman. We have found this idea woven into the attitudes, legal battles, and conflicts regarding many aspects of the emerging status of women. The gratifications of pregnancy and obligations to have children are used as arguments against contraception, abortion, the right to sterilization, and even the idea that a woman should have a unique identity of her own. For most women, this argument tips the scale in favor of keeping every pregnancy and raising every child. There is no way of knowing how many women keep every pregnancy because they want to or because they simply feel they should.

The Pregnant Woman Comes First. Of all the people who must consider the pregnant woman's status in the world, she has the absolute right to consider her own needs first. It is the quality of her life that is important and has the right to be most important. The quality of a woman's life does not mean the amount of ease and comfort she enjoys, as opposed to the amount of hard work and troubles that she may go through. It does not mean whether she keeps any particular pregnancy or puts it up for adoption or terminates it. The quality of each woman's life is explained by how she feels about herself and how she feels about the effects of her actions on her family, her loved ones, and her friends.

Who has the right to decide what is right in each pregnancy? Many people enjoy judging others but are not willing to pay the price by living with the results. But only the woman herself has the obligation, the right, and, indeed, the justification to make the judgment and decision concerning her pregnancy, and determine how it is to affect her and her world.

The only valid exception is the rare instance of severe personal incompetence, where there is no choice but to have a responsible person step in. The fourteen-year-old girl who had encephalitis at age three and whose mentality froze at that point, who clutched her doll and asked, "Momma, why are these people poking at me?" has little choice in this matter.

Most women, however, can understand quite adequately, perhaps through counseling, the implications of a pregnancy and its effects on themselves and the people they love. I must reassure these women that the choice must be theirs. Other people might try to make it for them, but only the pregnant woman herself lives with that choice. It is the certainty of a woman's decision that determines the quality of many of her relationships from that point forward, regardless of what she chooses. Every woman has the right to decide her life and her fate for herself.

The Family Factor. Many people, as I have noted, suddenly become part of a woman's thinking and consideration when she faces an unwanted pregnancy. But obviously, the woman herself is the most deeply involved of all. From the moment she discovers it, no woman can forget the potential of life within her. Anyone who suggests that this decision is made easily or thoughtlessly by any pregnant woman or by those close to her has had no contact with how these decisions actually are made. It certainly helps her if those around her care about her and her welfare first. She then has the freedom to choose what seems best for her.

Sometimes it turns out that families are the least able to help. Marion's parents raved about how nice it would be to have grandchildren even before she got married. Her husband turned out to be a very dependent man, and needed more of a mother than a wife. She knew it couldn't last. That meant there was no comfortable way to speak freely about how she felt to any of the three. She was quite torn in deciding what to do. Continuing the pregnancy might please everybody else, but simply letting it all happen seemed like an inescapable jail sentence of maternity. Had she not been able to confide in a close friend, she felt sure that she would have lost her mind. Carla, on the other hand, was Catholic. Unlike many other women of that religion, she could not be comfortable telling her husband or friends that she was pregnant and considering an abortion.

Fortunately, most of those who may be touched by the circumstances of an unwanted pregnancy *are* willing and able to put the woman's needs and feelings above their own.

Two things are not likely to change: The woman who keeps her pregnancy has made a commitment and assumed responsibilities that will last for many years. And the woman who decides to terminate her pregnancy has made a difficult personal decision that will never be altered. This is much easier to live with if she knows it was the very best decision she could make.

The Rushing Hand of Time. Most of life's problems can be put off, at least for a little while. Pregnancy allows no such luxury. Pretending it doesn't exist amounts to a very firm decision to bear a child. This doesn't eliminate the chance for a strong, healthy emotional environment for raising a child, but it doesn't make it any easier.

Teenagers should take a special warning from this. The fear of telling parents has to be faced sooner or later. Putting it off does not put off that unavoidable discussion. It is apt to lead to no choice at all, other than a youngster's having the baby and reducing a barely developed lifestyle to compensate for it. Parents should open up lines of communication at the very earliest stage of mature understanding so teenagers aren't afraid to talk frankly with them.

Preabortion Counseling: When Is It Important? Preabortion counseling is always important. It offers much more than a simple discussion of alternatives. It includes more than explaining the medical procedure and answering questions. It goes into depth about how a woman really feels in that moment of her life and how it affects everyone else. Whatever she chooses, this decision will always stand as a milestone, a moment when she faced a fork in the road and had to determine her fate. Preabortion counseling helps a woman solidify her decision based on what is right for her.

If this step is omitted, each reminder of an uncertain pregnancy can potentially reopen a painful wound instead of bringing a woman the comfort that she made the right decision.

I have spoken with many women who have endured the risks and uncertainties of an illegal abortion. I've spoken with many who have terminated their pregnancies in clinics in which individual counseling was not available. I've spoken with many who have had abortions in the offices of genuinely sympathetic gynecologists, or by their family doctors in a hospital. In almost all these cases one serious flaw appeared time after time. That was the ongoing, painful uncertainty of whether the choice was made with the most thorough of all considerations. *That uncer-*

tainty proved to be a deeper thorn over the years than the results of the decision.

In other medical decisions it is never assumed that a patient knows her problem and therefore can answer all the essential questions herself. This must never be assumed in decisions concerning pregnancy. If we are talking about treating a whole patient and not just her uterus, the conscientious availability of individual counseling does make a major difference.

Counseling goes beyond providing a woman long-range emotional security. It provides an extremely valuable opportunity for a professional to review the cause of each woman's problem so that it may be prevented in the future. This is much more than a sympathetic pat on the back and a prescription for contraceptives. Many pregnancies reflect a cry for help or attention from parents, a husband, or a boyfriend. The deaf ears of parents or a physician in the face of a direct appeal for contraceptives is another reason for the necessity of counseling. To help a woman see the cause of her pregnancy and explain to her the steps by which she can avoid it in the future requires, in most cases, a surprisingly short amount of time. Years of on-the-couch psychiatry are not usually needed. Trained and sympathetic understanding is.

This understanding reveals that at this moment, women need much more than to be slotted into a mass medical system that provides instant treatment. The patient who reaches for abortion because she is under severe stress but is inwardly leaning toward another alternative *must* be discouraged from having the procedure. My counselors have seen many, many women who came in for an abortion, but indicated during counseling that if their situation were somehow a little different, both they and the father of the pregnancy would rather keep it. In such a case, the counselors go into depth to help a woman pinpoint her balance, values, and desires in life, and then encourage her to go back and discuss the situation again with the man. At least some of these women, in this deeper final discussion, find a way to keep the pregnancy.

In the same way, a few women realize that adoption is better for them than the other alternatives. In these cases, they are referred to quality adoption counseling services. Under no circumstances should a physician or a clinic dealing with abortion have anything to do with controlling adoption.

In the end, about one out of every ten women who come to my clinic will carefully reconsider another alternative if given the chance to talk out their decision with a thoroughly trained and sympathetic counselor. The other nine who have an abortion are glad for having had one final chance to talk it through, this time with the reassurance that they have determined, with as complete confidence as possible, what is right for them. Not surprisingly, this makes a big difference in deep feelings for years to come.

The Personal Decision. Even after the rest of the world reviews the pieces of a problem pregnancy, it is still the woman herself who must put it all together. No one else can feel what she does, and no one should pretend that she or he does. It's like trying to understand someone else's pain. There comes a point where only the person experiencing it can know it.

Not every woman has difficulty in making the decision to terminate a pregnancy. Frequently, there is no realistic alternative.

Anna felt that she had little choice. She fit the molds and did the things that parents and teachers had always approved. She worked hard at her job both before and after marriage and two children. Her husband had a moderately good income, but a little more was always needed for their kids or themselves. The pleasure of making them happy with little unexpected surprises made the extra effort well worth it. She related to her husband, friends, and social groups the same way. The idea of intentionally upsetting anyone was totally foreign to her.

When her husband died in an auto accident, her children were in their early teens. At this worst possible time, she learned that she was pregnant again. Within only a matter of weeks, much of her world had collapsed, and the rest seemed destined to crumble in the future. From a logical standpoint, her friends advised, terrible as it was, having an abortion quickly was the only sane thing to do. Time was getting short before that twelve weeks' deadline she'd heard about, and a sense of urgency bordering on panic settled over all the rest of her misfortunes. The problem was that she wanted to do it, because in a way, it needed to be done. But then, here was the last potential living legacy of her husband, whom she loved.

In the evening, she looked at her children doing homework and watching television. They were hurt and missed their father. Being young, they learned to laugh again more quickly. Those sights and sounds were the only bright moments in many hours of staring at kitchen plates, crying silently in a bed that had grown much too large and cold, and waking before dawn in a desperate struggle to think clearly.

Even the woman in her bathroom mirror began to say, "For God's sake, your life is mangled up enough. You owe it to your children, if not to yourself." The woman in her bedroom mirror noticed what seemed to be a little bulge as she was getting dressed. It said, "How can you think of such a thing! You're carrying a life in there. Ted's life. You owe a lot to them both. What would *he* have wanted you to do?" The reflection in the hall downstairs brought another reminder. "Your watch. Look at your watch. It's later every second. Run!" She did just that, out the front door and into her car. She almost had an accident herself.

Her doctor had sympathized to the extent of agreeing, "Well, you really do have a problem," but offered little else. It seemed to come down to a choice of what was the right thing to do, since there was no good answer in any direction. She could think of only one place more. She didn't care what her minister might say. For sure, he'd say something. Whatever it was, she would do.

"I can't and I won't tell you yes or no," he said. "We speak so much about doing the right thing. It has to be right for you. Don't say that doesn't matter anymore. It matters because it's you who have to live and hopefully make life better for everyone else around you. The answer lies in how *you* best can manage. If you can make it with a third child without losing yourself or sacrificing the closeness with the other two, that's fine. If the best you can do is at the breaking point now, then you must save what you still have. The decision must be yours, because only you know these critical answers."

It wasn't the relief she expected, but his few comments did make sense. The next several days were an emotional roller coaster she'd like to forget. Out of it came the idea that what would be best for herself would be best for all concerned. They were not two different things pulling in opposite directions; they were really one and the same. She stopped looking over her shoulder at work, wondering who else knew about her pregnancy and forming opinions of what she should do about it. Even the women in her three mirrors began to fade.

She came to the clinic, and after going over everything one last time with the counselor asked, "I wonder how many other women go through what I've been through?"

What Are the Medical Abortion Procedures?

When a woman comes through the clinic, she learns that once her decision is made, the hardest part of terminating a pregnancy is over. The medical procedure is relatively simple, in trained hands. It usually takes between five and ten minutes, and can be likened to a moderate amount of dental work. A visit to a clinic may take three to four hours, however. The additional time allows for a pregnancy test, a pelvic exam to confirm the pregnancy and determine the length of gestation, counseling to discuss the decision and explain the procedure, the procedure itself, and about an hour to recover.

First Trimester. A first-trimester abortion is usually an outpatient procedure that is done under local anesthetic. This means that a woman does not have to be admitted to a hospital or have a general anesthetic, which puts her to sleep. A very small percentage of women do have medical or emotional problems that make the hospital approach of a general anesthetic advisable, but these are only a few percent. Most first-trimester procedures involve cramps that are similar to those of a menstrual period, but this is almost always over within an hour.

During the call for an appointment, basic information is taken and specific information is discussed. The call concludes with a set of instructions concerning clothing, who to bring or not, length of stay, the importance of having someone else do the driving, payment for the procedure, and directions to the facility. Suggestions are also made about eating and drinking before arrival, what to bring, and when a woman might resume her normal activities. Questions are expected. All of the information taken is confidential and cannot be released without consent.

On arrival, a receptionist completes the basic information on the chart. Then the pregnancy is confirmed with a test and its duration is determined in a pelvic exam. If there is any factor that does not match up between a woman's calendar date of her last period, the size of her uterus, and the pregnancy test, the doctor in charge will ask specific questions to determine what is really happening. At most clinics pregnancy tests and pelvic checks are offered free of charge whether or not a procedure is performed. If there are no problems in dating the pregnancy, standard laboratory work is taken, such as blood count, blood type, urinalysis, testing for venereal disease and so forth, exactly as is done in a routine hospital admission.

The results of the blood-type test are extremely important. Approximately 15 percent of all women have Rh-negative blood. If a pregnancy is Rh positive and the mother is Rh negative, then early Rh-positive blood cells from the pregnancy may get into the mother's bloodstream. This event does not hurt the mother, but it may harm a future Rh-positive pregnancy. There is a serum that should be given in this case. It has the ability to inactivate any Rh-positive material in a woman's blood before it conditions her system to make protective antibodies. These may react defensively against a future Rh-positive pregnancy. This serum is somewhat costly, but it is definitely valuable for most, if not all, Rh-negative women.

After the pelvic examination, most clinics offer counseling. This is a review of an individual woman's situation, problems, and decision, so that she may have the assurance of having made her best choice. This can be done in either group or individual counseling, but our experience has demonstrated that individual counseling works better. Both forms of counseling must explain the procedure so that the woman understands what will happen as well as rare but possible complications. Both approaches provide the patient with a consent form and the opportunity to ask any questions so that she may feel certain of her decision. This is standard practice for all surgical procedures, both large and small. It is in individual counseling, however, that a woman can usually face her situation with the greatest openness and honesty. It is in individual counseling that a woman's husband, boyfriend, or parents may join her in talking through the decision to whatever extent and for however long is necessary. It is in individual counseling that a woman can go into great depth about her feelings, values, relationships, expectations for her life, the problems that caused her pregnancy, how these problems might be solved, avoided in the future, and where to go or what to do for further help if needed. I believe that the best way to meet every woman's personal needs is to respond to her problems with thorough individual attention.

The best time to perform a first-trimester procedure is from the eighth through the twelfth week of pregnancy. In that interval the mechanics are easiest, success rate greatest, and complications least. Some facilities offer procedures for terminating pregnancy before eight weeks, the point of the second missed period. They call this "menstrual regulation," or a variety of similar names. I cannot recommend this practice because many women missing only one period have proven not to be pregnant at all. Of the ones that are pregnant, a significant percentage of procedures do not work because it is too early. Then the whole thing has to be done over again.

Premedication usually consists of a mild tranquilizer,

if anything. Some form of medication is generally a good idea because excessive nervousness or apprehension about anything, a medical procedure or otherwise, can make an unnecessarily large production out of something simple. It is neither possible nor necessary to pretend that a certain amount of emotional concern is not part of this moment. It is not even necessary to be completely at ease and relaxed, though certainly the more relaxed the better. If the staff of nurses, counselors, and medical assistants are sensitive and empathetic people, a light touch on a patient's arm, a reassuring smile, or open support of the patient accepts the woman as an individual and offers the warm understanding that she is among people who are helping her. The great key to this moment is knowing what is happening and having confidence in the decision and the directions of the doctor at hand.

Physicians and the nurses who assist them take the procedure just as seriously as the patient, despite the fact that they may have done many of them. Most of these highly trained people understand the emotional implications of this moment as well as the medical techniques. Many of them have the knack of transforming even the most difficult cases into relatively simple exercises with the help of personal interest, light conversation, and perhaps a touch of humor.

During a procedure the patient lies on a table in the same way as in any other gynecological exam, with her feet in stirrups. After washing the vagina, a local anesthetic is injected around the cervix, which is the entrance to the uterus at the top of the vagina. These injections sting for a few seconds, but are no different from any other shot. No one enjoys an injection of any kind, but the important message is that there is nothing more exotic or dramatic about it than a Novocaine or similar injection at the dentist's. There are occasional rare complications from allergy reactions, just as there are with any medication, but the overall safety record is excellent. In fact, the safety factor is much greater than with general anesthetic.

There is one important thing a woman can do to help her procedure go simply and easily. This is to let all her muscles be as loose as she can make them. Even while some degree of nervousness or emotional tension continues, it is possible to relax tense muscles. One to several deep, slow breaths can help this happen, if during these breaths everything is allowed to fall by gravity.

A woman's hands can be her guidepost. If she can keep her eyes open and concentrate on some object at the same time that she follows directions, and also thinks about leaving her hands relaxed, then all the rest of her muscles, including those in her vagina, will relax and this will prevent excessive discomfort. If a woman is trying to relax but notices that her hands are tightly closed or grip the side of the table, then she should open and relax them and this will immediately help relax the rest of her body.

After the anesthetic takes hold, the cervix is dilated, which means the entrance to the uterine cavity is gently opened. After this dilation, a cannula, or hollow plastic tube, is put through the cervix into the mouth of the uterus. It is connected to a small vacuum pump and a mild suction empties the uterus. An instrument called a curette is then passed around the inside of the uterus just to make sure, as well as possible, that no excessive clots or tissue shreds remain. The procedure is then over.

The entire process takes about five to ten minutes.

At that point, the patient is given a shot of Methergine, a medication that helps the uterus contract. If it is indicated, she is also given the Rh serum mentioned earlier.

In the recovery room patients respond better to relaxing in a reclining lounge chair than to resting in a bed. The release of the tension built up waiting for and going through the procedure, together with any residual cramps, gives most women a passing feeling of being quite exhausted. This generally lasts a very short time, usually less than fifteen minutes. As soon as possible, women are encouraged to begin moving about, and their strength returns rapidly. During this time, care is taken to make sure that there is no excessive bleeding or other signs of possible problems.

The first stage of recovery may contain transient nausea or dizziness as well. This is usually the result of overbreathing due to tension, or it may result from the dilation of the cervix itself. As a rule it does not indicate any significant difficulty. We recommend no eating or drinking before the procedure because of this tendency. One of the first sure signs of recovery is a very normal realization of being hungry. At this point light refreshments such as coffee, soft drinks, and cookies generally fill the bill quite well.

Thanks to the use of a local anesthetic rather than putting a patient to sleep, the transition from weakness to hunger to a strong impatience to return to friends or family or go home is quite rapid and dramatic. From time to time a common drugstore variety of pain-relieving medication is called for to help ease the cramping. Narcotics are neither required nor recommended. If discussing afterthoughts with counselors will be of further benefit, they are available. Afterthoughts rarely mean second thoughts. We see rapid relief and a readiness on the part of most women to resume their lives.

A very interesting phenomenon usually occurs during this time. In a moment of uncertainty, people react the way they think they are supposed to react. If even one woman out of four is bright, active, and positive, the other three are almost sure to respond the same way. If for some reason an atmosphere of quiet and heavy thoughtfulness is projected strongly by one woman, it's a good bet that all the patients will appear to be quiet, thoughtful, and relatively slow to respond. There are individual variations, of course, but the overall tendency to follow an upbeat note is so obvious that these clues have led us to take particular care in providing bright, colorful decorations and a slightly stimulating musical background. Like the friendly warmth of physicians and nurses during the procedure, the therapy offered by cheerful interior design has proved to be as valuable as any medication.

After being given prescriptions and postoperative instructions, most patients are discharged from the recovery area within an hour. Their experience generally proves easier and more positive than they had expected.

Second Trimester. The second trimester is medically and legally defined as extending from thirteen to twenty-six weeks of gestation. Most physicians take the option of not performing the procedure later than twenty or twenty-two weeks to provide a more than adequate margin of safety short of viability.

About 80 percent of second-trimester pregnancies are discovered only one or two weeks past the critical twelve-week point. A small number of gynecologists have expanded and developed a dilation and evacuation technique for early in the second trimester, similar to a first-trimester procedure. The advantages to the patient are a faster procedure and therefore a smaller expense. But most physicians still feel that the greatest patient safety lies in a totally different approach, because of the potential of excessive bleeding.

The usual second-trimester procedure is done in a hospital because of the medical need for patient safety.

The procedure takes an average of nineteen hours. Almost all of this time is spent in reading, watching TV, or sleeping.

It begins with an injection of medication into the uterus through the abdominal wall. Some people are frightened by this idea, but the technique is relatively simple in skilled hands, and once again, has proven to be little different from any other injection to most people. The injection removes some fluid from the uterine cavity and replaces it with medication.

This withdrawal of fluid is the same technique used in genetic testing during pregnancy to discover deformities when this tragic possibility exists. The physicians who have perfected the skills of second-trimester abortions are the ones who have become most deeply involved in this area as well. It is also possible to determine the sex of a pregnancy in this way. But despite the growing discussion of this subject, extremely few patients and even fewer physicians would seriously consider terminating a pregnancy simply because its sex did not conform to the patient's preference.

In an abortion, the medication is injected into the uterus through the same needle that withdrew the fluid. The kinds of medication used may vary. They include saline solution, glucose solutions, urea formulations, or prostaglandins. Each medication has its own advantages and disadvantages, as is the case for all medications, but they all produce the same reaction. They stimulate the uterus to contract and produce a miniature labor which discharges the contents of the uterus.

When this occurs, no operation is involved and no general anesthetic is necessary. The physician's skills are required to put the medication in the uterus, observe the patient for possible side effects, and evaluate her after the procedure to determine that she has come through it safely. When the procedure is completed, the patient is checked and, when ready, is discharged, to be followed with a postoperative checkup in a matter of weeks.

Three new techniques that have been widely used in second-trimester abortions are now being seriously studied for use in full-term pregnancies and deliveries. The first is the use of prostaglandins for stimulating normal labor. The second is the use of a tight cylinder of rolled seaweed called laminaria, which expands rapidly by absorbing great quantities of water, and may assist in the dilation of the cervix, which is necessary for naturally or artificially completing any pregnancy. The third technique is sonography. The sonograph emits and receives sound waves, which are harmless. The sound waves bounce off internal tissues and bones and paint a cross-section picture on a cathode ray screen, which resembles a small TV set. This is perfectly safe and has great diagnostic value. It may be used before a second-trimester procedure because it can determine the exact length of gestation with much greater accuracy than a calendar or even a careful pelvic examination can provide.

After the Procedure. The most dramatic thing about recovering from an abortion is that it is undramatic, simple, and routine. At least half of the women say something like: "I don't believe that's all there is to it. What else is there for me to do?" The truthful answer is very little.

After a first-trimester abortion most women are able to return home within an hour. Almost all patients return to work or school the following day, and I can recall any number of women who jumped right into strenuous activities.

Dominique, for instance, was a professional dancer who had finally won the chance to join a large show in a featured role. The only advice she needed to carry out her obligations was to take an extra capsule for cramps, to be sure to take a tablet to prevent excessive bleeding, and by all means, wear at least a couple of pads, because you never know when unexpected bleeding might develop. She called the next day to thank us for the advice and to share the good news that her first rehearsal was perfect.

Specific instructions after a first- or second-trimester procedure are simple, straightforward, and to the point. First, whatever medications may have been prescribed should be started immediately. These commonly include an antibiotic to guard against possible infection, and Methergine to contract the uterus and prevent excessive bleeding and some of the cramps, if any occur. My clinic's policy concerning pain medication has always been to avoid narcotics because they are not indicated. Most women do quite well with standard analgesic medications, plain aspirin, or nothing at all.

Two specific restrictions are important. A woman should not douche or have intercourse for at least three weeks, until after her checkup. The reason for this is to avoid putting anything in the vagina that might carry bacteria and thereby cause infection. By the end of three weeks, the cervix, which has been dilated, closes again and protects the uterus. Tampax can be used within two to three weeks with relative safety, but in the interest of greatest security, pads are best during this interval.

A frequent discussion in the recovery room reveals a lot of concern about the merits of postoperative bathing versus showering. In reality, there exists no hard and fast prohibition against taking a bath. Bathing itself does not float bacteria and subsequent infection in through the vagina. The greatest medical reason for favoring a shower is the very practical observation that it is impossible to predict the onset of unexpected heavy bleeding.

The most frequently asked question in the recovery area has little to do with any of this medical information. It is, "When can I wash my hair?" Through all my years of training and practice, I have never been able to figure out what the relationship might be between a woman's head and her pelvis, which is, on the average, at least three feet away. To resolve this question once and for all, let me offer this considered rule of thumb: If your hair needs it, then please, by all means, wash it.

Another question most women ask about a first- or second-trimester procedure is, "How will this affect my ability to become pregnant in the future?" The answer for both procedures is, "Absolutely no different than you might expect after a full-term pregnancy." Conception is possible again at almost any time after either procedure. Menstruation may resume anywhere from two to six weeks after either procedure and, on occasion, may take several months to be restored—the same as in a full-term pregnancy.

Complications: How to Recognize Them and What to Do. Complications of any surgical procedure may involve infection, excessive bleeding, or injury to part of the body. Most problems, including drug reactions evidenced by rashes or swelling, make their presence known within a few days and should be brought to a doctor's attention without delay.

After a procedure a woman's body reacts like it is recovering from a normal full-term delivery, but in a much smaller way. Any combination of spotting, bleeding, or clotting may or may not occur. Several days or several weeks may pass with no bleeding at all, and then several bouts of bleeding or clotting may be experienced. Most women simply have variable amounts of blood-tinged drainage for a month or more, until the woman's body resumes its normal menstrual cycle. At least once a day someone calls to say, "I'm not bleeding at all. What's wrong?" Little or no bleeding signifies no problem. Too much bleeding, on the other hand, should be reported at once.

There is a great deal of variation in the amount of cramps that may be experienced. Cramping is generally the same or less than a woman experiences in a moderately heavy period. Just as the majority of women manage menstruation with a minimum of fuss, so most women manage recovery from a procedure in the same way. Some have no pain at all and a few must take a little time off to rest in bed. Any extremely severe pain greater than anything a woman might experience in a difficult period should be reported to a doctor.

Infection is not common, but may be serious. The presence of a discharge does not necessarily indicate infection, and prolonged slow bleeding may be normally accompanied by an unusual odor. The true indication of infection is generally a combination of severe pain with a temperature elevation over 100.6 degrees. If a woman has any questions or symptoms on this point, a physician should be consulted to make a determination and offer any treatment that may be indicated. Life-threatening complications are considerably more rare than any of those mentioned. The most conservative published statistics indicate that the mortality rate of abortion is less than that of a full-term pregnancy.

Approximately one woman in four hundred needs to call a doctor for a significant problem, though calls for an explanation of symptoms—basically, reassurance that nothing is wrong—are common. All of these calls are important, because the confidence that everything is all right is an important part of recovering from any surgical procedure. Most problems are minor and resolve themselves. If there is a serious question, then a gynecologist *with experience in the field of abortion* should be consulted. He will determine whether or not further treatment is needed. A far too common reaction of many physicians unfamiliar with these procedures is, "Quick, let's put you in the hospital and do a D and C." Ninety-nine times out of a hundred all the fuss, expense, lost time, and exposure to additional medical procedures is unnecessary.

A woman's vulnerability to pregnancy is extremely high after an abortion. Contrary to the popular myth, the next menstrual cycle may begin within a matter of days, without a woman's having even the slightest indication that it is happening. Most clinics, including my own, prescribe birth control pills or another contraceptive directly following the procedure. When the pill is used, it regulates a woman's system and puts her right back into a monthly cycle.

Beginning the *immediate* use of some form of contraception is *always* advisable. Irregular periods or even the absence of periods does not mean that pregnancy cannot occur again. *Every woman in this position must be cautioned not to fall into the trap of taking her safety for granted, because the problems that led to her initial difficulties, in all likelihood, still exist.*

One final word of reassurance is important for both patients and physicians who have only a superficial familiarity with this procedure: *It is possible for a pregnancy test to remain positive for up to six weeks after termination of pregnancy.* This fact must be stressed because of the many apprehensive phone calls I have received from patients and physicians alike running premature postoperative checks on the procedure. Chances are a thousand to one that the procedure worked well. This reassurance should spare both patients and physicians many anxious moments.

Three Weeks Later: A Physical Checkup. A follow-up exam after this procedure is important to make sure that everything was successful and that there aren't any complications. It consists primarily of an adequate pelvic evaluation. The patient also has the chance to ask any remaining questions.

The physician consulted need not be a gynecologist on the staff of an abortion facility. He does not even have to be a specialist in gynecology, so long as there are no major problems. The choice of physician or facility may be a matter of convenience, expense, or personal preference.

By this time, every woman has had the opportunity to consider the effects of an unwanted pregnancy and to plan the prevention of future problems. This generally, but not always, involves the use of contraception or sterilization.

About one out of twenty women rejects the idea of birth control and won't even acknowledge that she may need it at all. It is not the job of a physician or clinic staff to harass any woman who has had an abortion into submission on these points. It is important to realize that this woman, if she is bent on repeating her problems, may need specialized help. She should be told in no uncertain terms that the door to this help is open. That's all that can or should be done, but in these cases it must be offered routinely.

Finally, access to ongoing communication should always be extended. The experience of putting all the pieces back together begins in the recovery room, and it may not reach a resolution in three weeks. Women should be invited to ask for whatever additional guidance they may need. So many of them are surprised to learn of its easy availability.

Who, When, and Where?: Finding the Best Doctor, Clinic, or Hospital

One of the cornerstones of the movement to legalize abortion was the fact that the critical nature of an unwanted pregnancy led it to be terminated without even the hope of safety. The days of the back-alley abortion, the horrors of the coat hanger, catheter, knitting needle, or, at best, the midnight haphazard procedure in a sympathetic doctor's office are almost gone. These ended too often in the emergency rooms of major hospitals, which dealt routinely in shock medical attempts to preserve the lives and bodies of helpless victims. Those who fought for safe, legal abortions genuinely believed that if they could accomplish anything to preserve the emotional stability and lessen the painful scars of the woman and the people in her world, they would have produced a miracle. Today, most couples have recognized and appreciated the deep personal meaning of the new, compassionate maturity of law and medicine.

This miracle is still in its infancy. There are excellent clinics available today, but there are some that should be guarded against. In my most sincere medical opinion, regardless of the causes of an unwanted pregnancy, it should only be terminated in a facility that provides the best possible medical and emotional care.

When a woman or a couple has a problem, what can they do to secure the best possible help? Basically, make several intelligent phone calls and ask specific questions to determine which local facility provides the highest quality care, according to the standards we have researched and developed at my clinic.

All of the following questions can be asked and the answers evaluated by the patient herself, together with her family. Direct questions on the following points to any clinic listed in the phone book are not only acceptable but intelligent. The highest quality clinics are delighted to have the opportunity to discuss or explain their services to any prospective patient.

Who performs the procedure? The procedure should be performed by a physician trained in the specialty of gynecology. If he is an M.D., he should be board eligible or board certified by the American College of Obstetrics and Gynecology. If he is a D.O., a doctor of osteopathy, he should be certified by the Osteopathic College of Obstetrics and Gynecology. Certainly, he should be fully licensed in the state in which he is practicing.

Where is the procedure performed? A first-trimester procedure may be performed in a hospital, a physician's private office, or an outpatient clinic. Neither of the first two choices is ideal. Simply having a procedure done in a hospital can triple its cost without offering a proportional increase in safety or emotional concern. Hospital personnel are, in the main, untrained in the specific emotional and medical problems of pregnancy termination.

I do not favor the practice of offering a first-trimester abortion in a physician's private office. The procedure itself is relatively simple, but it is not *just* another procedure. As in a hospital, a physician's office lacks adequately trained personnel from either a counseling standpoint or a specialized medical treatment standpoint. Many private offices, even the ones engaging in a moderate amount of outpatient surgery, are not equipped with the emergency backup equipment that should be present in the event it is needed. For this procedure, emergency equipment spans the range from oxygen and intravenous solutions to defibrillation apparatus (the heart "shock" machine needed in the extremely rare event of cardiac arrest) and emergency medications that are specific to this procedure. In addition, many private physicians who perform abortions in their offices administer intravenous medication that produces almost total unconsciousness, similar to a general anesthetic. They do this to offer "an easy experience." The problem is that this medication, in my opinion, invites complications rather than avoids them, without offering any significant advantages to the patient.

The best alternative is an outpatient clinic specially set up and equipped to handle the emotional and physical problems of abortion. These should be selected carefully, however. Not all clinics are alike.

Is an R.N. available? When the procedure is performed, the physician should have the assistance of at least one graduate registered nurse, and possibly an L.P.N., a licensed practical nurse. These people are well-trained assistants capable of being of great value in any possible emergency.

Are there lab facilities? In searching for the best available service, it is proper to inquire about the presence of adequate routine laboratory facilities, including the capability of administering anti-Rh serum.

Is there personal twenty-four-hour assistance for individual problems? In the event that a patient or her family has any important questions or problems, can she contact a physician on a twenty-four-hour basis at any time after the procedure? The concern and commitment of the physicians involved is sometimes apparent in a clinic's answer to this question.

Is there ALTERNATIVE counseling? Inquiring as to the availability of *trained* alternative counseling is another valuable question. No physician or medical facility should perform any form of treatment, most especially an abortion, if a patient does not understand all of her alternatives and chooses the solution that best suits *her* needs.

Is there INDIVIDUAL counseling? Deciding what to do is the most complicated part of dealing with an unwanted pregnancy. One sign of the quality of every clinic is the adequacy and competency of its counseling. A self-styled amateur who plays at counseling may cause as much mischief as an irresponsible medical student who plays at surgery. For example, an emotionally troubled sixteen-year-old was brought to my clinic by her mother, who was herself under a great deal of pressure. This young woman's pregnancy test was negative but her pelvic exam showed indications of pregnancy as well as an abnormal pelvic mass. The counselors at my clinic spent a great deal of time with this young woman and her mother and came to the conclusion that the youngster subconsciously wanted to keep the pregnancy in retaliation for her mother's necessary restrictions on her social life. They also concluded that the young woman's latest boyfriend was taking advantage of her self-destructive tendencies. He had neither the desire nor the ability to help in the pregnancy or after it. In good faith, I referred this young woman to her own gynecologist for the specific purpose of having her pelvic mass evaluated since she might need long-term follow-up. In an act of totally inexcusable irresponsibility, he let his receptionist discuss this girl's problem as if she were a counselor. This "counselor" caused irreparable harm to both the young pregnant woman and her mother. By the time this amateur was finished, none of this young woman's alternatives made any sense to her. The waters of her mind had been muddied beyond belief.

A few dozen more stories like this immediately come to mind. The lesson in all such cases is that counselors should be *trained*. They should have a degree in a field

of human relations. They should also have in-service training and experience in the field of abortion counseling.

The offering of *individual* counseling is more than a
nice gesture on a clinic's part. It is a strong indicator of
the sincerity of concern for the individual patient and
reflects the high level of quality and medical care that may
be expected. A reasonably intelligent secretary or an office
nurse can be trained to memorize a list of important questions and give the appearance that she knows what she is
doing. *This superficial training is not adequate for recognizing psychological danger signals and the need for referral and professional help, or at least additional in-depth
alternative counseling.*

In my clinic, for instance, counselors may advise
against having a procedure if they feel the patient cannot
handle it for any of a wide spectrum of reasons. Counseling lasts for as long as each patient needs assistance with
her decision. When each patient's turn comes, at that moment she's the only person in the world.

Is there GROUP counseling? Group counseling may
be conducted as well. It consists of one counselor talking
about the problem of an unwanted pregnancy to five or
six women at a time. In the best of circumstances, it provides each patient the feeling that she is not alone. Like
group therapy, group counseling has many strong sup-
porters who feel conscientiously that it can work. In my
opinion, it may only represent a shortcut of time and expense. Considering that the entire basis of legal abortion
is a medical response to an individual need, then individual counseling speaks for its own importance.

Is counseling open to others? Are the others involved
in an unwanted pregnancy—boyfriend, parent, husband,
friend, or minister—permitted to join in the counseling
session? If they are, they should enter the discussion after

the pregnant woman, by herself, has had a chance to discuss her own situation and her own feelings with the counselor.

Is there postabortion counseling? Postabortion counseling should also be available. The primary reason for all this emphasis on the function of counseling is *not* to make anyone's mind up for her. It should help a woman find peace with her decision *whatever it may be.*

What is the ideal facility? The ideal facility for a first-trimester procedure is a clinic ,(or a clinic outpatient service attached to a hospital) specifically designed to handle both the medical and emotional needs of women at the least possible cost. Upon investigation by phone, a quality facility should provide satisfactory answers to the great majority of questions that have just been reviewed.

Is the cheapest procedure the best? Price alone should never sway a decision, even though many patients have financial difficulties because of their age or family obligations. A difference of twenty, thirty, or even fifty dollars from one location to another should be secondary to the other considerations that determine the medical and emotional quality of the care.

It is true that almost all facilities require payment in advance for the procedure because of the unpredictability of insurance carriers under any circumstances. Most insurance companies consider an abortion part of their benefits, but there are many companies that routinely work at getting out of claims of all kinds. It is also an unfortunate fact of life that some patients compel this requirement because of the way they abuse credit. Without a "pay in advance" policy, many clinics would not be able to exist and still meet the needs of patients at a reasonable cost.

How to find the best place. Referral to a clinic that has a long-standing, excellent reputation can generally be obtained by asking local health departments, county medical societies, obstetric and gynecology societies, or any random selection of two to three reputable gynecologists in the area. Clinics themselves are usually listed in the phone book, but the largest notations often do not indicate the most reputable clinic.

Advertisements for this medical service that appear on radio, billboards, or television frequently illustrate the *lack* of quality since advertising practices of this kind reflect, rightly or wrongly, a disregard for what is considered to be good medical ethics in most, if not all, communities in this country. Any facility that disregards this fine point of medical ethics may well have disregarded some of the other, more important aspects of it as well.

Many social crisis agencies provide good information in this area. These are often excellent services and may have names like "Hotline," "Crisis Intervention," and so forth. Where a valid Planned Parenthood agency is operating, it may also provide objective, reliable recommendations.

Any agency that exists for the purpose of abortion referral alone, and charges a fee for this service, must be considered highly suspect. Many states have outlawed referral agencies entirely. The same caution is true for agencies that attempt to channel a woman into the process of having a baby and then putting it up for adoption, unless it is a recognized, reputable adoption service. When there is *any* question, the validity of any and all of these referring points should be checked with a local chamber of commerce, medical society, or Better Business Bureau.

When a woman needs a second-trimester procedure, the answer to questions concerning the best hospital and the best physician are generally found easily from the people who make the most frequent referral to them, the most reputable first-trimester facilities. There, she should also insist on a detailed discussion of her individual case, an explanation of exactly what is involved, and a thorough, professional consideration of the alternatives.

Any clinic, hospital, or physician who offers this procedure but practices less than total dedication to every patient's needs fits my personal definition of an abortion mill. That description has nothing to do with the volume of cases performed. No one would call an optometrist's office an eye-glass mill. A mill implies the haphazard spewing out of less than first-class work, whether in one case or many thousands.

Abortion was only recently legalized and standards for quality performance are still emerging. The word *mill* still applies to many sources of abortion when there is a lack of motivation to put the patient first. This is demonstrated when the full range of medical services, emergency safeguards, and the unique emotional needs of every patient are not satisfied. In my view, the private office performing a few abortions a year, the general hospital bending its availability to permit a dozen or so procedures a year, or the clinic that does thousands of cases but offers only a loose form of group counseling may deserve the description "abortion mill," if these facilities do not provide for the patient's physical and emotional needs in the best possible manner. Every woman, every family, and every concerned person involved has the right and obligation to ask questions, look into these points, and seek the best care available.

5
WHO ELSE CAN HELP?

A pregnant woman's final decision about whether to keep her pregnancy must reflect *her* needs. She is the one who has to live with that decision, no matter what it is, for the rest of her life. To be right for her it must be made by her. Others around her might think that she ought to be happy, that what has happened to her is wonderful, or that she ought to be punished and made to feel terrible. No matter what they think, they can add suffering and grief to the pregnant woman if they don't support her in what she feels. Whether she feels her pregnancy is wonderful or a tragic mistake, the people close to her should help her deal with her situation in terms of her honest feelings.

Husbands and Lovers. The moment a woman tells the father of her pregnancy that she is pregnant, the next sixty seconds shows the whole story. His emotions and reactions tell more about the depth of his relationship and concern than any words he may ever use. His reaction may be the determining factor in the woman's deciding whether her pregnancy is a blessed event, something to make the best of, or a tragedy in her life.

Seldom does a man step onto such a stage. His every expression, emotion, and feeling has an overwhelming impact on his audience of one. His feelings may well be a shock and a surprise to himself. He has no opportunity to think about a "proper" answer. This kind of surprise may not always be pleasant, but it does bring out sincerity of reactions.

All the circumstances in a relationship may seem to be terrible, but a man may be simply delighted at the announcement of pregnancy. If that is the case, his first reactions may well prove that what a woman feared was a problem is not a problem at all.

If a relationship appears to be wonderful on the surface, but a man's reactions are defensive or threatening, he has confirmed that a severe problem exists. Whatever further thoughts, plans, or excuses he may make, those first sixty seconds may convince a woman that if she keeps the pregnancy, this man may offer her and her child less than adequate support in the future.

Sometimes there is very little choice. A fifteen-year-old young man who has managed to get a fourteen-year-old teenager pregnant is hardly in a position to be comforting or wise. The same may be true of a twenty-eight-year-old man who has been kidding himself as well as a woman into thinking that a really worthwhile, lasting relationship was in the cards. A husband with no chance to increase his income and barely able to support a wife, several children, and a mortgage may react less than romantically if the pregnancy represents nothing more than another intolerable stress.

Reactions that are totally unreasonable and emotionally dangerous also occur. A relatively small but noticeable number of men are openly hostile at the idea of supporting a woman emotionally, financially, or otherwise, and at the same time put the entire blame for a pregnancy on her. They present the distorted logic that since the woman was responsible she should be punished by keeping the pregnancy. Exactly how everything might work out is her problem.

The amazing thing is that there are many women who still fall into the pit of taking this irrational nonsense seriously. One of these women, Francine, explained it by saying, "I still love him and there's nothing else I can do."

Fortunately, most cases at my clinic show that the most common male reaction is healthy and helpful. The man demonstrates concern and offers the woman his support in the framework of the reasonably solid relationship they share. Whether the pregnancy is kept, terminated, or adopted, it is the sincere concern of a man for a woman's welfare and well-being that is likely to have a positive effect on their relationship and the woman's feelings about her decision for the rest of her life, regardless of the decision she makes.

Parents. No matter what the age of a pregnant woman, whether she is in her mid-thirties or a young teenager, whether she is married or single, no matter what her circumstances, a frequent desire is to *not* involve parents. There are two main reasons for this. First, most women feel like Pam, who was twenty, that she must take the responsibility to sort out her own problems.

This isn't always possible. The younger the woman, the harder it is for her to exclude her parents. She is simply dependent on them for her physical and emotional support. The very young teenager may have no option at all, but her desire *to protect her parents* is still there. This is much more common than the motivation that might be expected: the fear of punishment for getting pregnant. The phrase "I can't tell my parents, they'll just destroy me" is heard occasionally. The explanation given by Renée, a totally helpless fifteen-year-old, is much more frequent. She said, "I can't tell my parents. They have enough to worry about and this will just tear them up."

There is a second reason why parents are not included. Too often, they and their daughter have never become real friends. A lack of meaningful communication is not the cause of this unhappy situation. Frequently, it is the result of it.

Friendship is not a question of permissiveness. It is the quality of relating to people as they are, rather than as they might be or should be. Parental friendship does not interfere with the desire to help or the setting of limits within which a child must live. Limits set by parents for children may or may not be severe, but the children who live within them make a judgment of their own. That is the realization and comforting feeling that their parents are sincerely interested in their well-being.

With a teenage woman, more often than not the girl's parents and the parents of the boy who made her pregnant are brought into the situation. Their initial reactions are likely to be defensive. The girl's parents may take their child's physical maturity as a personal insult. Or, the pregnancy may be seen as a symbol of their failure or the child's rebelliousness. These feelings are understandable, but they are generally inaccurate. A teenager's personal relationships do not come about in spite of the quality of home life or the sincerity of the parents' efforts. They come about because each child, growing into adulthood, reaches out to develop a world of her or his own.

"That's great," one father said when we discussed this, "but does it have to extend to getting pregnant? We certainly didn't raise her like that. It had to be her boyfriend's fault." But that boy's parents didn't raise him to fool around and get girls pregnant either. Each family wants to feel that the other kid's delinquency, rather than their own teachings, played the major role in producing this serious problem.

But how much *teaching* has there really been in either family? How much did these parents really talk to their growing children about the business of sex and the problems it can cause? Did they explain to them the rightful enrichment of a relationship that it can bring, under even half-reasonable circumstances? The one failure which many parents in this situation must accept is the failure of deep communication.

That failure is frequently laughed off with, "What the hell, my kids know more than I did at their age. I feel silly lecturing them about the whole thing." That excuse may well be true. Parents in their thirties and forties are often less comfortable about sex than their own teenage children, but if they don't have perfect wisdom at least they have the advantage of experience. They have seen good and bad relationships in their own lives and in the lives of many others. This is more important wisdom than their degree of comfort with sex. It is the knowledge of how to recognize and prevent problems that should be transmitted with protective directness. The sharing of these experiences may open a door through which a young woman or a young man can walk and get help when she or he has a problem—*before* the problem becomes a catastrophe.

A frequent and reasonable question at this point is, "Fine. All this is great before the kid became pregnant. But how am I supposed to react now that she is?" Again, reaching into a parent's own personal experiences provides the most valuable guide.

All parents in this position should ask themselves, How would I like to have been treated if I had been faced with an unexpected pregnancy when I was a teenager? What kinds of attitudes in my parents would have helped me through that hassle? Would my life have been better or worse if I were branded a degenerate, or if I were given no help and understanding? How would I have felt if someone tried to make my decision for me and forced me into it? And don't forget the last important point: Would I have wanted to be helped to prevent another pregnancy six months or so down the road?

Thinking through these questions might not solve all of a parent's concerns immediately, but they do provide a very good place to start. They give each parent the ability to identify with their child's troubles. That identification will help if parents want their child to reach *her* best decision, not force her into their own mold. According to the maturity, intelligence, and age of a pregnant young woman, that decision may be any of the three choices: adoption, abortion, or planning to keep and raise the child.

Offering sincere help and friendship is easier than most parents think. Children may grow up faster than before, but their emotional needs are the same. They want reassurance and approval. They want a sense of satisfaction that they have not hurt others by their decisions. If a young woman can be helped to make the choice that leads to the least amount of harm for her and the others in her world—including the children she might want under better circumstances—more than half the responsibility of parental involvement will have been completed.

More often than not, the rest means allowing the young people to walk through the doors of their decision with enough personal dignity that they gain more self-confidence to continue making responsible decisions in the future. They must be granted enough independence and adulthood to openly communicate with others and benefit from the guidance of both professionals and their friends, since their overall problem is really that of becoming mature and responsible adults.

With a little luck, this situation can improve a family's relationship. The young woman or the young man can gain two trusted adult friends, rather than wind up having to live with two hostile parents.

Friends. In an unwanted pregnancy, true friends of both the woman and the man are valuable possessions, indeed. Friendship means liking someone as they are, within reasonable limits. It is close to the idea of receiving pleasure from seeing another person happy. This happiness is not a momentary wild enthusiasm, but another person's well-being over many years.

When a friend is in trouble and comes for comfort and advice, then friendship becomes much more than a pleasant relationship for amusement. In this crisis, one friend can give another the vital assistance of sincere interest, confidentiality, and enough objectivity to review an entire problem thoroughly.

First, friendship becomes a sacred bond in which the interests and needs of the person requiring help are put in a position of the greatest importance by the person who is helping out. That sounds easy enough to do, but it takes careful thought and a willingness to give, sometimes, it seems, endlessly.

After sincere interest, the second ingredient in friendship is confidentiality. Unless a friend in trouble is on the verge of seriously hurting herself her privacy should never be betrayed. If a friend chooses to share a crisis, this decision was made with the expectation of confidentiality. This point is important. A problem pregnancy is sometimes revealed to people who yield to the mischievous temptation of painting the person in trouble into a soap opera, then stepping back to watch the show.

Objectivity is the third kind of help a friend can provide. Most of the time, people have the experience and intelligence to evaluate their problems realistically. But when a person pounds her brain past the point of endurance, she becomes a victim of too much thinking. Then a devilish reaction called negative feedback sets in, and every time a specific thought comes to mind it is immediately balanced by a reason why it may not work. In other words, every time a decision is planned, it is immediately blocked by a reason for rejecting that decision. Logic gets lost on a merry-go-round. A gust of fresh, clean objectivity provides reassurance that one decision is indeed reasonable.

Objectivity is also a safety check that helps prevent a foolish and perhaps harmful conclusion from being reached. This does not mean making the decision for the person with the problem. But it does mean helping her find her own best decision, and then, if she needs it, assisting her in carrying it out.

Once a decision for abortion is made, small but valuable amounts of assistance may be required. This may include helping with the driving to and from the clinic, shopping for medication, or baby-sitting for one day. These may seem insignificant, but what the woman receives is much more than that. Family and friends who show that they care and give sincere support, during and after the experience, offer the most meaningful gift anyone can give.

6

THE HELP OR MISCHIEF OF PROFESSIONAL GUIDANCE

One of the most important things a woman needs is a sounding board for her judgment. The comfort that comes from the warmth and genuine interest of others helps so much in any stressful situation that requires a major decision. A woman with a problem pregnancy may be able to get valuable help and reassurance that her thinking is clear from the people who are close to her.

If the people around a woman cannot offer her the essential ingredients of sincere interest, confidentiality, maturity, and objectivity, she may turn for professional advice to her doctor, a counselor in a clinic, or others who might offer reliable assistance by virtue of their training and experience. *This is the reason for any appeal to professional help and advice.* As long as the needs of a woman are respected and put first, then that professional assistance is a great and gratifying gift for one human being to give to another.

Physicians. A physician is more than a technician who saves someone from heart failure or removes an occasional appendix. Most of the time a physician does offer all of the virtues of objectivity, sincere interest, mature judgment, and experience. These are tall orders but they are practiced in most instances by the men and women who dedicate their lives to their profession, despite the press of time and commitments.

Unwanted pregnancies and abortion present special difficulties, even to concerned physicians. The medical and mechanical aspects of this subject are relatively new and may not have been included in a doctor's training. The emotional issues are frequently much more complex than those a physician deals with during an average day. The greatest difficulty physicians experience is the lack of time to go into the personal depth required.

If a physician does want to help, he or she must apply the best objective judgment to a specific individual's problems. The physician does not have to be intimately acquainted with all the fine points of the procedure or all the emotional aspects of abortion. Every physician has seen patients suffer from problems beyond their capacity to cope, and this degree of experience and compassion will help. If unable to do at least this, the doctor should be honest enough to explain his or her own limited exposure or adverse personal attitudes in this area and refer the woman to a professional who can handle her problems. Patients who have enough personal dignity to have put their faith in approaching a physician deserve no less than this. In addition, they have the right to test each of the keys mentioned in accepting or rejecting the physician's counsel.

These statements are presented strongly because I have seen so many examples of physicians who have violated the trust given them. They ignored a commandment of professionalism: the obligation of objectivity. They trampled that obligation by placing their own emotional needs and interests above those of the patient, the person coming for help. As a physician with respect for that title, I am offended by any example of such transgression.

During the course of writing this very chapter, a couple was referred to me by a reputable gynecologist. Virginia was a twenty-nine-year-old Catholic, faithful in spirit as well as attendance. Her husband, Ken, was no less dedicated, and they had two children and very much desired a third. She had an attack of abdominal pain and visited her family doctor, who in turn referred her to a general surgeon. Her symptoms were not clear and he had her admitted to the hospital for complete X-ray studies including a barium enema with fluoroscopy to check the lower bowel. This procedure introduces one of the heaviest doses of radiation to a woman's pelvis of all X-ray diagnostic studies.

Virginia missed her next period and assumed it was related to the stress and discomfort she had. When she missed her second period, she went to her gynecologist. He examined Virginia, came up with a positive pregnancy test, reviewed the history of her exposure to radiation, agreed that there was a strong likelihood of her having an abnormal baby because of this, but went on to command her to have the baby anyway because that was her duty. If her fate was to suffer through the anguish of such a pregnancy as well as whatever horrible results might be produced, then that was Divine Will. It was not her place to question it.

Good religious training notwithstanding, it was all her husband could do to keep from attacking him on the spot. He knew instantly that regardless of the outcome, this man who abused the title "physician" had scarred his wife's peace of mind for the rest of her life.

Ken could not let the matter rest and went through a nerve-racking search for at least one honest opinion from a physician who might be both competent and fair. Calling friends and associates for suggestions, he felt like the wanderer in an ancient Greek parable looking for an honest man. One name came up several times and he took his wife for a consultation.

This doctor realized the depth of this couple's emotional and physical problems and contacted a professor of radiology from a nearby medical school to verify the seriousness of the facts at hand. He himself did not feel comfortable with the idea of performing an abortion because of his own ambivalence on the subject, but he did counsel this couple fairly and referred them for the procedure if *they* came to the conclusion that this was their best alternative.

Whether a physician's guidance involves abortion, tonsillectomy, or removing a pimple, his advice carries neither the responsibility nor the necessity of trying to make up someone's mind for them. The role of a doctor who is intellectually honest is to acquaint a patient with the material facts of a problem, and to recommend and review courses of action in light of potential benefits weighed against possible risks. These statements may seem so obvious that to mention them may be offensive. No offense is intended. This reminder should not injure the sensitivity of physicians who practice in good conscience. Those who have forgotten these simple precepts and thereby cause overwhelming mischief deserve to feel outraged, but they should direct their hostility where it belongs, at themselves.

Psychiatrists. After gynecologists and family doctors, the next group of physicians most involved with the intimate aspects of abortion are psychiatrists. These professionals were initially brought into the picture after the legalization of abortion for the purpose of routine consultations. Hospital boards and medical staffs responded to their own programed attitudes that the primary reason for the existence of any woman is to produce babies. Therefore, any woman challenging this premise, regardless of her circumstances, had to be somehow emotionally disturbed. This whole process carried the subtle indignity of implying that no normal woman could envision the need for terminating a pregnancy. This was a sham and a rip-off, and psychiatrists themselves were the first to object to being so used. Certainly, cases did exist of mental incompetency, severe emotional stress, trauma from rape, and harmful pregnancies that upset the delicate balance many a woman or her husband needed for emotional stability. The great majority of cases did not fit these categories, and most psychiatrists recognized this to be true.

One young woman who was treated by two different psychiatrists comes to mind. Marlena was a fourteen-year-old tomboy, physically well-developed, with good intelligence but poor stability. Her need for attention extended beyond any amount of praise or affection her parents could give her. She took an almost sadistic delight in commanding their full attention by a succession of acts with an increasing degree of shock value. She started the hobby of caring for snakes, enjoyed exploding firecrackers, smoked cigarettes and pot whenever she could find them, and began running away from home and disappearing when she was supposed to be in school. Next came her visit to the clinic, where she dramatized the thinly veiled threat of becoming pregnant. We discussed her problems with her parents, but before anyone could do anything she turned up in an emergency room after having swallowed a fistful of sleeping pills which she had obtained from someone in school.

This last act threw her automatically into the hands

of a psychiatrist who happened to be on call for emergency service that day. He shared something with his newly acquired patient: a reputation for dealing with life through sensationalism. Part of that posture he expressed by being a supermoralistic enemy of abortion. He was not impressed with the unmistakable call for help in this girl's history. Instead, he was totally preoccupied with probing her sexual fantasies and lecturing her on the virtues of keeping the pregnancy, which seemed destined to appear on the near horizon. His approach was based on impressing her with the evils of abortion and explaining to her bewildered parents that this was essential so that she could learn about life the hard way. Taking care of the results of a pregnancy was supposed to make her a stronger and better person.

Yes, this episode really happened. It was unprofessional, not because of an individual physician's own philosophy. It was unprofessional because of the absence of objectivity.

Marlena's parents recognized that they were being misled and took their child-woman to another psychiatrist. He was concerned about the real threat of potential pregnancy as well as the threat of attempted suicide. His approach was to review the day-to-day effects of these potentially harmful actions, then formulate alternatives that might more successfully meet Marlena's needs. At no point did his personal feelings about the advisability of abortion, adoption, or keeping the pregnancy enter the fabric of his counseling.

Medicine's most delicate balance is between providing help or doing great harm. That balance becomes even more precarious in new areas where physicians have little direct experience, specifically counseling related to unwanted pregnancies. I make a plea for objectivity because it has to be made. Any physician or other professional connected with this problem must keep in mind the highest precept of medicine: "First, do no harm."

The Clergy. Many women avoid looking for help from priests, ministers, and rabbis because they fear a negative moral judgment. They feel that theirs is a realistic problem of day-to-day existence, and a clergyman may turn it into an abstract discussion that will upset them more than it will help. As a result, one basic concern is often left unanswered: "If I take this step does it mean that I have to consider myself an immoral person for the rest of my life?" Many women find a reassuring answer to this question within themselves. Others must look further.

The childhood religious background of some women may be so strong that they need to discuss their feelings about their personal image with a clergyman—his position symbolizes moral judgment. It is not accurate to suppose that most women with problem pregnancies have no religious feelings. Nor is it accurate to suppose that most religions refuse to recognize the needs for abortion. In fact, the reverse is true.

The growing list of religious organizations that have taken a position in favor of legal abortion points out that most religions recognize strong and legitimate needs for this procedure. Some of these are listed in the Appendix, and include religions such as the Baptist, Lutheran, Methodist, and Presbyterian churches. No blanket approval by them is implied or intended. Under ideal circumstances, women who require help in adjusting reality and religion may emerge from a conversation with their ministers with greater emotional dignity than they expected.

It is true that circumstances are not always ideal. Rhonda's case was a difficult one. She became pregnant in the midst of a divorce. The problems that led up to that point built slowly over many years and could not be reversed. She had two children in elementary school and was prepared to support them when the final papers came in. A pregnancy was the last thing she could manage at that time. The whole sequence of events made her more upset than angry. She would have liked to have another child if it were possible under decent circumstances.

She called her husband and asked to meet him. She really tried to be as gracious as possible and salvage both the marriage and the pregnancy, but it never happened. When her husband learned that she was about three months pregnant, he became furious. His own plans for what he wanted to do and with whom were falling neatly into line. Going back again with even greater responsibilities presented him with all the excitement of being dragged to jail. "Why didn't you tell me you went off the pill?" he stammered. "That's just another perfect example of how stupidly you do things."

Rhonda believed that her most reasonable course was to terminate the pregnancy. She thought about how far apart her and her husband's lives had drifted, and that the agreement on a divorce had come just in time to prevent bad fights from turning into violent ones. Her sister strongly disagreed and constantly dropped by and called, pressing the point that she could work everything out. Finally, her sister convinced her to meet her minister. She had spoken to him at great length, explaining that the only problem seemed to be that Rhonda didn't appreciate the importance of keeping everything together regardless of what personal sacrifices might be involved.

In his talk with Rhonda, the minister did not mention abortion much at all. He spent most of the time reviewing the ideal sides of marriage and the pleasant and positive aspects of raising children. When Rhonda spoke about her reasons for leaning toward divorce, and that, in fact, her divorce was inevitable because continuing with or without the pregnancy was an intolerable situation, she fully expected little more than condemnation for not trying harder. Instead, she was overwhelmed. The minister pointed out that he recognized the ideal and hoped for the ideal. He felt that everyone should put forth their best efforts toward the ideal in every situation. But when that ideal proves to be impossible, as was the case in Rhonda's marriage, morality spoke for the course of action that could salvage the most good. The discussion turned toward the relationship between practicality and morality. The minister embarked on a deep, sincere effort to help Rhonda find the course of action that was compatible with both.

Many women have reported that their faith in their individual religion has been strengthened or weakened when their minister showed whether he himself believes the words that sound inviting every Sunday morning. The minister who speaks of love but shows little compassion, love, or individual interest fails the test of his own words and detracts from the validity of his teachings. He suffers more injury than losing the trust of a woman. He loses a great measure of credibility for his entire philosophy. On the other hand, the clergyman who demonstrates belief in his own words and actions will have done more to strengthen a woman's faith than a thousand sermons. I have heard these thoughts expressed many times by women who have taken the option of keeping a pregnancy or putting it up for adoption, as well as those who elected to terminate it.

Social Workers and Psychologists. These professionals offer a degree of insight into the depth and various aspects of individual problems. They can also act as a fail-safe buffer against the pitfall of grossly distorted judgment.

By the time most women appeal for professional help they are more interested in reassurance for the soundness of their thinking than in having someone make a decision for them. The words they use may not indicate this attitude. However, when a patient says, "I just don't know what to do," she really means, "There are so many sides to my problem, I want to make sure I'm reading the scales correctly." Every counselor's number-one question, "What do you *want* to do?" proves this point more often than not.

The responsibility of objective professional judgment can never be written off lightly. One couple in their late twenties explained that they had a difficult time arriving at the decision to terminate the pregnancy, but they came to the clinic because it seemed advisable. They had a whole list of reasons. The more they spoke the more it became apparent to the counselor that they really preferred to keep the pregnancy, if this, that, or another factor were slightly different. The counselor was impressed by their concern and exhaustive searching. She felt they were hoping for the reassurance that they might be able to make it with this pregnancy after all. The interview was far from a short session, and the ultimate decision was to manage with the pregnancy.

Why did this couple come to an abortion clinic to review their decision instead of an agency programed toward keeping pregnancies? They wanted to have the benefit of what they considered the most severe test of their feelings. This approach may sound foolish, but it demonstrates a mechanism of thinking that many people have.

On rare occasions we see the reverse of this. Kim, a single twenty-two-year-old, went to an agency whose stated purpose was to preserve every pregnancy. I don't know the exact words she used, but they carried the message, "Help me punish myself for being such a miserable, stupid woman." Telltale hesitation cuts on her wrists were easy clues that this woman had been suicidal, and that her appeal was clothed in a serious emotional cloth. The counselor recognized the need for a psychiatric interview, and Kim took her recommendation. She came to the clinic with the realization that she was using her pregnancy to hurt herself because of deep problems for which she had begun receiving treatment.

Counseling for an unwanted pregnancy is specialized, and the great majority of social workers, psychologists, and their assistants have had little direct exposure to these comprehensive yet specific "moment of truth" reviews. Without doubt, advice can be given for any problem, but it is easy to misinterpret symptoms and signs that indicate difficulties. If a case is complex, it must be referred to a source where adequate information and insight are available.

Public Health Workers. Workers in public health departments see a great volume of requests for abortion, family planning, and sterilization. They have helped patients time and again with sound advice and referrals. They have also had the opportunity to evaluate the results of those referrals. Experience with these problems has given them, in general, the ability to make knowledgeable recommendations for further counseling or whatever a woman may require in the way of responding to a pregnancy, whether it be keeping it, adopting it, or terminating it.

The biggest limitations are bureaucratic, not personal. Many counselors and nurses in public health departments have been severely limited by directives or stipulations from their immediate superiors. They have been told what they are and are not permitted to discuss. The subject of abortion is still a controversial, "hands off" issue to many bureaucrats who have never seriously investigated the problem and have no personal exposure to it.

A tragic reality faces people in the front lines who are trying to provide care to those who need assistance the most. These directives and limitations are for the most part tied to fears of losing budgetary allowances. Someone further up the government money chain might be antagonized. It's unfortunate that the higher the source of policy and financial authority, the further it is removed from the actual problems of patients.

Many nurses and social workers in health departments almost routinely place their jobs in danger by assuming personal responsibility for discussing problem pregnancies with patients who desperately need guidance in some direction. The cases are generally not dramatic and do not make wonderful magazine articles. The problems are simple and often tedious to the average listener because they come wrapped in the bleak realities of everyday survival under difficult circumstances.

"What am I going to tell this girl?" Brenda, a county nurse, asked me. "Should I tell her that she was just foolish not to keep up with her daily birth control pill and send her back on the street? What can I say other than that she won't qualify for this or that assistance program? If I get my boss's feelings right, I'm supposed to give her a lecture implying that she is personally responsible for everyone else's higher taxes. At the same time, I'm supposed to tell her that she might be better off keeping the pregnancy rather than terminating it, despite the fact that she has no support at home, and, if she has the child, no one to turn to except welfare. If I try to suggest my boss's favorite alternative, would you tell me how to make a convincing pep talk for adoption while I'm wondering how many people want to make a nice home for a little black baby?

"Really helping this woman is worth the risk and frustrations," Brenda said, "because I wouldn't feel I was doing my job right any other way. If I didn't have to worry so much about getting in trouble for being honest, though, my job would be a lot easier."

Nearby Helping Hands. There are a large number of people with varying degrees of experience who provide fringe medical care. These include nurses, crisis line volunteers, school counselors, teachers, and even medical office secretaries. They share in common a general awareness of the kinds of problems people have and the chance to be of great assistance in the realization stage of any crisis. Their contribution, over many years, has led to a sense of public trust and a respectful public assumption of their interest, dedication, and professionalism.

The fact that they are on the periphery of providing service offers comfort to many people who may begin the search for advice without making a commitment to an authority who is prepared to take action. This informality makes these first discussions especially valuable.

The relationship of informal trust also carries a notable pitfall. Nurses, crisis line volunteers, teachers, or other nonspecialists concerned with unwanted pregnancies may exceed the limits of their information and training in responding to questions that may seem simpler than they actually are.

I have learned of many cases in which an office nurse or medical secretary took it on herself to expound her opinion of when, where, and how a pelvic examination or pregnancy test should be done, and under what circumstances a termination should or should not be considered. It's important to realize that there may be strong legal, social, occupational, and even patient dangers in yielding to the temptation to substitute personal opinion for hard medical facts, or for the lack of being able to recognize the danger signals of someone's overreacting to great stress. To a woman under severe pressure, the words of an office assistant may be taken with the same authority as those of the doctor who employs her. This oversight can lead to a great deal of trouble.

The best suggestion is to remember constantly the necessity of referring women who need help to the best possible sources of information and assistance as gracefully and rapidly as possible.

7
RETURNING TO NORMAL

Emotional Recovery

Weeks of turmoil have been compressed into a matter of hours of final decision, medication, undressing, dressing, moving from one place to another, passing a blur of faces, and enduring a few minutes of unfamiliar sights and sounds. The coiled emotional spring then unwinds and a process of expansion begins, with a strong sense of direction established in the recovery room, confirmed in the first return to friends and family, and defined over the next few weeks. Within this length of time, a woman may redefine her life. At this point, the good or bad of abortion is interesting but not really significant. Of real importance is each woman's unique attitude and relationships with the people who played a part in her experience.

Coming to Terms with the Experience. In the recovery room, one young mother sits quietly with her eyes closed and her hands folded, considering how her infant children might react to her if, when grown, they learn of the problem she has had. Another, with a few strands of hair graying at the temples, leans forward on the edge of her lounge chair, determination on her lips. She is secure in her world and secure with her husband. She must immediately take steps to prevent this nonsense from ever returning to their life. A nineteen-year-old secretary is alert and chatty. The pregnancy was no fault of her own. Her IUD simply did not work. Her concern over this experience is no less than the other women, but she has the knack of handling heavy experiences with a light touch and the self-confidence to carry it off. A thirteen-year-old has almost no expression at all. She just sits there in a torn blue sweater and a thin cotton dress, staring straight ahead, one sock up to her knee and the other halfway down. The nurses and counselors come by to say something nice, offer her a drink, try to get through. She is polite, says very little, and then speaks only with her eyes. Her mother sits with her and explains that she has been like that ever since the attack —they never did find the boy.

At some point in the recovery room as many as half of the women cry. Their eyes overflow with emotion, sometimes relief at being able to live a normal life again, sometimes in the pain that marks their individual passage through this experience, sometimes from the anxieties they feel for the future. Will the world be kind? Will the world be better? What changes must I make? Even more, what changes are waiting ... out there?

The first few minutes of returning to the waiting room and seeing friends and family answers most of these questions. If ever there was a second chance for a husband, boyfriend, parents, or a close friend to solidify a relationship with warmth, that greeting in the waiting room provides it. Feelings of love or hostility, caring or annoyance, acceptance or impatience, make a lasting impression. To the woman, that impression stands for the rest of the world. No put-on works. No words are important. Only the simplicity of undeniable, real feelings determines the quality of this moment.

It's so much easier for a woman to return to and deal with her world when she feels capable of managing herself. It's so much easier for her to manage herself if she has the security of at least one person who really, really cares.

Returning home is nothing like the free-swinging brawling of a midafternoon soap opera. It is a quiet, slow, and deep process. The most reassuring observation I can offer is that, overall, the world changes very little despite the significance of anyone's personal crisis. For the most part, an accident of nature is accepted as just that in the eyes of the people who really count in the life of most women. Having gone through this experience may or may not contribute to making her a better person. Most certainly, this experience will not contribute to making her any less.

Your Relationship with Your Husband or Boyfriend. When coals are shaken they glow more brightly and their shapes can be more easily seen. When a husband or a boyfriend reacts to a serious problem in a woman, the strength or weakness of his real feelings stand out brightly. In a pregnancy that is wanted or even tolerated and made the best of, the kinds of problems that try the sincerity of a relationship under really adverse conditions simply do not exist. In the first weeks after an abortion, the kind of feelings and patterns that are formed are of even greater significance than those leading up to it. The relationships that survive and grow usually do so from a foundation of personal strength and affection, because these elements were present to begin with. Those that fall by the wayside in the course of this experience may cause pain, but in their loss their true deficiencies are laid bare. If they were made of such flimsy stuff, they probably could not have lasted anyway.

The crucible of this stressful experience melts out redefinition and reevaluation of many sides of a woman's life. Annette didn't want to be a strong, independent woman but it always seemed that people relied on her before she had the chance to reach out to them. After a while, her attempts to reach out became stiff and awkward and even more uncomfortable than before. Her pregnancy was caused by a man she felt sorry for. She wanted to comfort him and felt that if this was to be one of her roles in life she ought to do it well. The abortion jarred her back into a chilling sense of reality. She didn't want to be the mother of both an infant and a grown man at the same time. Her parents and friends were sincere but she saw little point in bringing them into her problem. Her biggest difficulty in recovery was deciding how to no longer insulate herself from the warmth that other people seemed to find in the world.

Theresa wasn't really sure of herself or the way other people thought of her. She was pretty and bright. Everyone seemed to know these things, everyone except her. It was almost as if a pathetic sickness haunted her. That feeling of never being quite sure sapped the strength out of so many experiences which should have been positive and memorable. When she found herself pregnant the thin platform of her own evaluation of her place in the world cracked in yet another seam. Her husband had always made her feel as though he deeply cared and wanted to build her up. Even on the way to the clinic, he said all the right things. Was it all a show? Was it the proper last expression of his obligation? Would he still be there next month, or, for that matter, tomorrow? These were the things that ran through Terri's mind. This merry-go-round of doubts had begun turning weeks before. It kept going faster and faster. There was almost a jolting sensation when the nurse led her from the recovery area back to the waiting room. It stopped. With the look on her husband's face, it stopped. She knew he was real. Months later, she dropped a note to her counselor to say a word of thanks and tell her that things were working out well. They had spent a very long time talking about that merry-go-round. She just knew that the counselor would remember. This time she was sure. And this time she was right.

Parental Return to Normalcy. Abortion cannot help but alter the relationship between a still-dependent young woman and her parents.

Recovery to an adult woman amounts to confirming the strengths or weaknesses of the various relationships in her life. Most often these are predictable. Recovery to the parents of a recently pregnant teenager means rapidly evaporating hopes of return to normalcy, the way things were, or, ideally, the way things should have been. The problem is that the old road is closed forever. The normalcy of relating to just a little girl has disappeared. If a solid road back to a loving home is to be traveled at all, it must be built quickly and *by the parents*.

Regardless of what emotional reactions may have come and gone, a new road of at least mini-adult recognition must clearly be offered immediately. It may be clear and inviting. It may lead the way to an overdue mutually mature relationship that can gain strength and depth through the years, leading to happier anticipations of visions of grandchildren. If it remains muddled in doubt and accusation, the inevitable result is to push a daughter further out of reach.

Her recovery is largely dependent on the reactions of her parents. That is why they must give the clues to the reassurance of their affection and sincere interest in her real welfare. Her response to those attitudes is generally positive, rapid, welcome, and relatively easy for her to achieve. That statement does not represent wishful thinking. I have seen it happen often.

The process of emotional recovery is deep and profound. To the degree that a woman receives help or pain from the people in her life, so she changes her reactions. Consider these moments of truth. Glenda's parents and boyfriend stood by her through her decision and procedure and left not the slightest trace of doubt about the sincerity of their interest in her welfare. Dolores, on the other hand, was stamped as nothing but an ungrateful, rotten kid who didn't have brains enough to know better.

Whether teenager or adult, the love a woman receives may affect her feelings about her relationships for years. Lucille was a woman who learned a harsh lesson about caring. She was tricked into pregnancy through the lie of a vasectomy. Shirley was told by her boyfriend, "You should have been more careful. It's your problem, not mine." But Nina, who was always on the brink of exhaustion from taking care of four kids and a house, was suddenly overwhelmed by the care, concern, and help of her husband, who realized that she was the most important person in the world to him.

It is not difficult to figure out which of these relationships are most likely to be weakened and which have the greatest probability of being strengthened by the truths brought to the surface in an abortion.

Postabortion Counseling: Indicated If Questions Remain. The fact that a pregnancy had to be terminated is unpleasant, and may have been a cause of emotional upset. More often than not, the need for an abortion is a symptom of underlying difficulties which may or may not be serious.

Most of these can be identified, understood, and dealt with by a woman so that they will not recur in the future. If there was misinformation about or misuse of contraception, that can be corrected easily. If there was a lack of adequate communication between a teenage woman and her parents, that might be improved. If there was a confusion about contraceptives being related to promiscuity, then a little clear thinking can go a long way. If there was a relationship that was deep but not secure, the test of a pregnancy may point toward more care in the future. In situations like these, which are the majority of cases, a woman's daily life can become more secure and rewarding if she comes out of this experience with greater personal insight and strength.

A minority discover that the circumstances of their lives deeply trouble them. For them, the problems that led to their need for abortion are not resolved with the procedure itself, even with the best of medical and emotional care. They may need further professional help. Assistance can be found in quality postabortion counseling.

The Reevaluation of Sex. Parts of our heritage still support the ideas that the primary value of a woman is childbearing, that sex is bad, and enjoyment of it is no more than the perversion of immoral people. When scrubbed clean of millions of words of argument accumulated through the ages, the way these statements have affected people stands out clearly. I have seen too many women in my obstetrics practice, as well as those recovering from abortion, interpret the stress of their experience as rightful punishment for their having enjoyed a normal relationship.

Marian's problems were a case in point. "I don't know what happened since my abortion," she said, "but I just don't feel interested in sex anymore."

"It's only been a couple of months. Are you worried

about getting pregnant again?" I asked.

"No, not really," she said. "I trust the pills pretty much."

"Do you feel any different about your husband? Are you upset with him for any reason?"

"No, he was just wonderful throughout the whole problem. If anything, I feel closer to him than ever."

"Did you enjoy sex before your abortion?"

"Well, kind of. I never thought that much about it. It felt good from time to time, but, mostly it was something I had to do. It made Fred happy."

"Didn't it ever make you happy, too?"

"I guess not," she said, her eyes downcast. "I'm not sure it's supposed to. Now, things are worse. The whole idea gets me upset and I wish he wouldn't bother."

Tonia, on the other hand, had a very different reaction. "Has everything gotten back to normal?" I asked during her three-week postoperative checkup.

"Yes, oh, yes," she exclaimed. "We've both done a lot of thinking about it. We went over everything five times and I think we're more sure of each other than we've ever been."

"Do you have any problems or questions?"

"No, except, I'm afraid we didn't wait for my checkup. Is that all right? I hope we didn't mess anything up."

"It doesn't look like you've done any damage but, out of curiosity, why didn't you wait? Did you miss it all that much?"

"A little, but I'll tell you, that wasn't the biggest part of it. We just wanted to make each other feel good. We have something wonderful to share. I'm sure that sounds silly."

"Tonia, don't worry about a thing," I had to tell her. "You should have waited, but you're in better shape than you know."

Most women think of sex as a normal, healthy part of life and they return to that conclusion fairly easily when they are involved in a sincere, warm relationship. They know that sex has two functions, both of which are valid. The first, of course, is having children. That is biological. The second is nothing less than the deepest and most personal form of communication, the giving and sharing of one's self. If a woman's attitude is such that she is at peace with both aspects of sex, her reevaluation can welcome it as a strong and healthy return of total communication with the man she loves.

Contraception: The Dangers of Confusion

The search for the perfect way to prevent pregnancy has been going on for thousands of years. Ancient Egyptians inserted a mixture of honey and spices into the vagina. Primitive Africans made a hole at the base of the penis so that most of the ejaculation dribbled out before entering the woman. Roman soldiers were issued sheaths of lamb intestine for use as prophylactics. There have been innumerable guesses at the cycle of female fertility based on everything from the length of rainfall to the phases of the moon. The Arabs are credited with the idea of the intrauterine device, or the IUD. They put flat pebbles into the uterus of female camels and this prevented pregnancy—in the camels. The origins of this discovery are unknown, but the first comment of a nomadic Arab father looking in anger and puzzlement at his teenage son must have been, "You did *what?*"

The Least Effective Contraceptives. There are four main kinds of contraceptives in use today, based on their effectiveness. The least effective category of birth control is the sincere expectations that often turn out to be little more than dreams. These are the pitfalls of the intention of abstinence, withdrawal, and the rhythm system, which are discussed in "The Great Maternity Trap."

Mechanical-chemical Contraceptives. The next step is the sexual tribal ritual of using something mechanical or chemical immediately before or after each experience of intercourse. It takes an unusual amount of will power not to skip using these methods of birth control from time to time, and this compounds the risk of pregnancy considerably. At best, these amount to an intermediate category of effectiveness. For instance, there is douching after intercourse. Even women who have douching paraphernalia loaded and waiting at the ready are lulled into a false security. The swiftest woman sprinter cannot get to her douche before a large number of sperm swim into her uterus.

On the other hand, teenagers have been known to shake a bottle of Coke into their vaginas at any number of odd locations with the same thought in mind, and the same lack of effective protection.

The use of foams and jellies reaches the 80 percent range of protection. This obviously is not ideal, but it certainly is better than anything mentioned to this point. These preparations also have the advantage of easy availability because they do not require a doctor's prescription.

The most frequent failures of these contraceptives occur because of improper use. It is vital to use a foam or a jelly before intercourse, and to use *an additional application* before every subsequent insertion that might lead to another male climax. Unfortunately, the bother and progressive lack of sensation sometimes outweigh these precautions. Also, regardless of physical annoyance, a woman should not douche for at least eight hours after relations if she uses foam or jelly.

Prophylactics (rubbers, condoms, etc.) are also in the 80 percent effectiveness range. They have the same advantage of easy availability as the jellies and foams. There are three main reasons prophylactics fail to work. First, they may break during intercourse. Second, they are used by many men after a preliminary penetration but hopefully before ejaculation. A third problem results from the idea that after an initial male climax is achieved with a prophylactic, the following insertions are safe without one. This is not true.

The primary value of prophylactics is for contraception, despite the printed announcement at the base of most issues: "For prevention of disease." This inscription amounts to little more than an effort to appease people who, for religious reasons, are not supposed to use contraception. Presumably, couples could pretend that they are preventing disease and not worry about pregnancy with a clear conscience. In fact, prophylactics may or may not prevent any kind of disease. If there is any real cause for concern in this area, it might be wise to wait for a better day, *after* a quick medical checkup.

Homemade substitutes for prophylactics must also be advised against. For a long time the microbopper set has been using cellophane and now Saran-Wrap. If someone has sense enough to bother at all, he or she should use a real contraceptive.

Diaphragms with jelly enter the 90 percent range of effectiveness, which is the highest reached by a mechanical contraceptive. The diaphragm has a potential place in the life of a relatively organized woman who can plan her sexual activity with a moderate degree of accuracy. The main drawback of a woman's going through the tribal ritual of inserting, positioning and checking the device before use is that her partner may become too impatient to wait, or, simply fall asleep.

The greatest reason the diaphragm fails is because it isn't always used. Other reasons for its failure include improper positioning over the cervix, the presence of a hole in it, the use of an inaccurate size, or being lost or destroyed when needed. As a woman grows older, the size required for a diaphragm may gradually change. It sometimes changes rapidly after the delivery of a full-term baby.

The IUD: An Effective, Easy-to-use Contraceptive. The IUD and the pill are the most important new developments in birth control. Other than sterilization, they are the first truly effective contraceptives available. They are also aesthetically pleasing, long-term contraceptives. This makes them a good choice for couples who enjoy sex spontaneously and don't want to worry about where and when it will occur.

The IUD is 97 to 98 percent effective. It offers the advantages of no effort in use and no intrusion during lovemaking. Once it is in place it requires nothing more than being checked about once a week, simply to make sure it is still in place. That is done easily, by feeling the fine thread left at the top of the vagina.

The copper and hormone-containing IUDs do require changing to maintain theoretical effectiveness. I have not become convinced that their advantages make the use of these types worthwhile. Questions in these areas should be resolved by each woman's doctor.

Some forms of IUDs are apparently safer and give better results than others. It is difficult to present a totally comprehensive survey on the subject because of many statistical variables that are impossible to pin down. Some of these are the exact numbers of IUDs inserted and the degree of proficiency of the physician in using proper size and inserting the IUD itself. At the clinic we have conducted an interesting study of 15,000 consecutive patients, recording the incidence of IUD failure. These findings are presented in the Appendices of this book.

Occasional cramps or spotting are not always indications that anything abnormal is happening, but should send any woman experiencing them right to her doctor for a check. These symptoms, by themselves, do not always mean that the IUD should be removed. There is no currently recognized justification for a physician's recommending a rest from most nonchemical IUDs after any time interval whatsoever, so long as it is working and does not produce significant problems for a woman. Questions in these areas must be answered by each woman's doctor. He has the responsibility of not overreacting to a complaint which the patient herself does not consider significant, and not recommending removal at the slightest provocation. This frequently observed overreaction all too often has led to an unexpected pregnancy.

The Pill: The Public Has Been Confused. At the present stage of medicine, pharmacology has made great progress in attempting to provide its own four freedoms. These are freedom from pain, freedom from infections, freedom from transient stress, and freedom from pregnancy. The last one came in the form of the birth control pill, which opened the door to many changes, attitudes, and healthy realities for women.

For the first time in history, women by the millions have the opportunity to assume personal responsibility for determining when they will and will not become pregnant, and can accomplish this vast change at reasonable expense, great availability, and relative safety. When used properly, the reliability of the birth control pill is over 99 percent.

The greatest threat of an unwanted pregnancy arises when a woman stops using the pill in panic for reasons that are not likely to be valid, and fails to insist that her doctor provide her with another form of contraception. This fear-prodded loss of the pill's protection causes many more times the numbers of pregnancies than does forgetting an occasional pill or two. Certainly there are cautions regarding the use of the pill, but these must be presented in the entirety of the pill's total safety record and perspective.

This subject must be discussed in depth because the growing national fear of the pill is damaging the public health far beyond any benefits it may receive. This problem is so vivid even at the level of my own clinic that it is overwhelming. Every single week pregnant women come to my office saying that they and their husbands or boyfriends have been frightened away from continued reliance on the pill because of one article or another. *In the vast majority of cases, careful review of the woman's history and physical health indicates that she demonstrates no specific reason for abandoning the pill other than fears which have never been substantiated by a doctor.*

So many of these unwanted pregnancies could have been avoided with even a small amount of reliable information from a physician. But, to make matters worse, many physicians have been intimidated by valid questions drawn from this, that, or another source. Physicians have recommended discontinuing or "resting" from the pill without giving or even having a specific reason. To compound the problem, these actions have been taken without specific alternate contraception being prescribed.

The net effect of the confusion about the pill has not been massive benefit to patient safety. It has been a swelling of the ranks of women with unwanted pregnancies, who are forced to run the far greater risks of physical complications and emotional pain that may accompany that condition.

Let me make an unequivocal statement to help

women in doubt put fears to rest in one often repeated area of nonsense and confusion: In my studied opinion there is no justification, without a specific medical reason verified by a doctor, for a "rest" from the pill, and there is no specific time limit for using the pill that has ever been acceptably demonstrated. Over 50 million women a year use the pill in apparent safety. The pill is without doubt the single most liberating breakthrough for women in history.

While it is important to be aware of the valid serious side effects that do exist, it is equally important not to overlook the overwhelming significance of this reliable contraceptive. In maintaining and supporting women's self-chosen lifestyles, freedoms, and abilities to engage in social and economic roles other than motherhood, it does all this with easy accessibility and greater safety than has ever been available until this generation. The pill also prevents the higher risks of abortion or keeping a pregnancy when a less effective form of contraception fails.

For those who don't know the overall picture, it is important to review both the harmless symptoms that may be recognized by a woman using the pill and the dangerous medical circumstances that may make the pill inadvisable. This is neither secret information nor is it difficult to understand. It is provided here for easy reference, and it includes responses to the most important questions that women ask.

In general, birth control pills are combinations of female hormones which imitate a miniature pregnancy on a month-to-month basis. The slight increase in hormones that circulate in a woman's body is much less than what is present in the course of a real pregnancy, but that small amount is enough to prevent ovulation, the release of an egg from a woman's ovary. Each ovary has the potential of producing thousands of eggs. Being on the pill for one year does not mean, for example, that there are twelve more eggs yet to be used, thereby extending the time of fertility beyond the menopause. At this time, there is no accepted evidence that birth control pills have any more effect on the menopause than pregnancy, which is no effect at all.

Because these hormones are similar to the ones in a normal pregnancy, some women recognize symptoms associated with pregnancy. These may include a tendency to fluid retention, moderate weight gain, changes in appetite, skin texture, pigmentation, hair consistency, and even breast changes. Sexual interest may increase or decrease on a transitory basis. Some women feel better and more vibrant than ever before. A small number experience episodes of depression. Many of these developments represent existing personal tendencies which may be *accentuated* by the pill rather than *caused* by it as totally new effects.

During the use of the pill, it is not necessarily abnormal to experience spotting and occasional cramping. Most of the time the reverse is true. Greater regularity of menstruation as well as less menstrual pain and less intermenstrual cramping are benefits of the pill praised by the majority of women. Unexpected bleeding without an adequate physician evaluation is not a cause for automatically discontinuing the pill.

Whenever the pill is discontinued, its use should be ended under the supervision of a physician, just as when it was started. Otherwise, abnormal bleeding may occur, and there may or may not be a delay in resuming regular periods. In general, the pill should always be discontinued at the end of a total cycle. The impulsive tossing of a half-used packet of pills into the wastebasket is *never* a proper method for ending its use. Occasionally after discontinuing the pill, it may take several months before normal, regular periods are resumed. Until that time, irregular bleeding or the absence of bleeding does not mean that a woman cannot become pregnant. This is true just as in the same interval after an abortion, a delivery after a full-term pregnancy, at the start of menstrual life, during the approach of menopause, or any time in between. A sexually mature woman may become pregnant without expecting it at any time before true menopause with or without a regular menstrual pattern. This has to be stressed because there are so many misconceptions about it.

There are specific reasons for not using the birth control pill, to be sure. Obviously, the most common is the simple desire to become pregnant. There are no currently proven bad effects on a pregnancy that occurs after the pill is discontinued. Birth control pills should not be taken during a pregnancy because of the possibility of masculinization of a female fetus and the possibility of subtle heart defects. The likelihood of a pregnancy while taking the pill properly is very, very small. However, if a woman on the pill suspects that she might be pregnant, she should check with her doctor immediately.

The second most frequent reason for ending the pill are cases in which the side effects—nausea, irritability, spotting, darkening of facial hair, and so forth—outweigh the benefits. Complaints of this nature are reasonable. Whenever the treatment of any problem becomes worse than the disease, another treatment must be found.

The third most frequent reason for discontinuing the pill involves a woman's realization that she *never* wants to have another pregnancy under any circumstances in the future. The age at which this kind of realization takes place has been dropping steadily over the past several generations and now seems to average out at around thirty. At that point there is a likelihood of seventeen to twenty or more years of fertility. That is a long time to visualize taking any medication, birth control pills or otherwise, and sterilization procedures may well be seriously considered.

Last but not least, there are some medical reasons for not using the pill. These are best diagnosed by a physician and not by a woman herself. If a woman has any suspicions, worries, or anxieties, she should see her physician instead of automatically assuming that prompt discontinuation is necessary.

The most important medical reason for not using the pill is an indication of a change in the blood-clotting mechanism. There are enough studies to suggest that there is significantly greater incidence of blood clots in women who have been taking the pill than in those who have not. Current evidence indicates that the risks of blood-clotting problems associated with the pill disappear when it is discontinued, regardless of the length of time of usage.

There are several other medical reasons for discontinuing the pill. The first of these is the presence of breast cancer. *There is no evidence that birth control pills cause breast cancer.* In fact, it has been shown that women who use the pill have less breast cancer than those who do not. However, it is possible that the pill may make an existing tumor worse. Acute liver disease is another reason for avoiding the pill, because the liver must process estrogen. However, any woman who has had problems with her liver in the past, but whose functions have returned to normal and are stabilized, may or may not be approved by her physician to use the birth control pill. The presence of strokes is a reason for not using the pill because one cause of stroke is problems with small blood clots. Several studies have been done on possible relations of birth control pills to heart attacks, but the results are not conclusive. Because of subtle changes in blood chemistry, there is a possibility that the pill may accelerate a diabetic process. Evaluation of this possibility must be made on an individual basis between a woman and her physician.

It has been suggested that women past the age of forty seriously consider other forms of contraception or sterilization than the pill. The reason for this thinking is that several of the medical conditions that make the pill inadvisable tend to occur with greater frequency after the age of forty. The most important thing to realize about these comments and suggestions is that they are no more than that—comments and suggestions. They are made on the basis of broad generalities and only a particular woman's personal state is important in this regard.

On the other side of the medical coin, the pill is used for a variety of reasons other than birth control. It helps many women correct painful periods, irregular periods, abnormal bleeding, some skin conditions, difficulties with internal bleeding, and cases of benign breast problems such as cystic mastitis.

To gain perspective, realize that there are some 50 million women using birth control pills every year. Regardless of what they read or discuss, these women enjoy both effective contraception and relative safety. There is no absolute proof that the pill causes cancer and it does not cause a delay in the menopause. That is the good news. What is the bad news? In the very rare case it may cause death, just as any other medication may. But how bad is bad? Birth control pills are safer than a multitude of commonly prescribed medications, ranging from antibiotics to medicine for heart failure.

In terms of relative risk, car accidents account for twenty-seven deaths per hundred thousand people. Pregnancy, overall, is responsible for sixteen deaths and abortion is responsible for three deaths per hundred thousand. There has been attributed only one death for every one hundred thousand users of the pill, and even some of those cases bear careful questioning. This set of figures shows that an abortion is about five times safer than a full-term pregnancy and using the pill is seventeen times safer than pregnancy.

It is my sincere hope, now that these facts have been put on the record, that the responsible media will see the public is sufficiently informed. The problems caused daily by the confusion over the pill must be corrected.

Sterilization: The Emergence of a New Right

If a woman uses contraception and it gives her a new kind of independence, from what has she been liberated? From a concept that has guided women's lives for centuries: that the primary purpose of a woman is to have babies and a primary responsibility of the rest of the world is to encourage her ability to do so. Today, that attitude has ceased to be universally acceptable. Our standards are changing. We can now choose our own identities, goals, and roles, whether we are a woman or a man. The ideal society at the end of this road offers genuine freedom of self-determination.

Most women enjoy feelings of gratification at the prospect of having a family, where and when they choose it. Beginning about a century ago, women gained the right to choose *with whom*. During the past generation contraception has begun to offer every woman the choice of *when*. Within the past few years legalization of abortion has provided, for the first time, a safe and increasingly comfortable choice of *when not*. At the present moment we are resolving the next major question, the woman's decision of *when never*.

Changes are coming about, but they are slow, and resistance to them is still very much in evidence. The woman who has had all the children she wants and decides that she simply does not want ever to become pregnant again may still run into major obstacles.

As usual, the government is the slowest to respond to the individual's needs. If a woman is receiving government support she may have to go through a long hassle of paperwork and evaluation and even have to obtain statements from doctors indicating that a sterilization procedure is absolutely necessary for preserving her health in order to have the expenses for this procedure covered. Legislators and administrators in government know that the cost of a tubal ligation, for example, is much less than the cost of a full-term pregnancy, and infinitely less than the cost of raising an unwanted child. Government resistance to support for sterilization has nothing to do with real economics. It's a hangover of the attitude "Babies forever."

Private insurance companies are a small step ahead of the government. Some of them have slowly and steadily broadened their outlook and support for individual needs of sterilization, but a great deal of resistance is still easily found.

The medical community is still far behind many women's personally expressed needs in this area, but many doctors must be congratulated for their progress toward realistically evaluating individual sterilization needs. Fading echoes of the philosophy "A woman's fertility must be preserved unless there is absolutely no choice" still vibrate through medical school classrooms, hospital corridors, and the offices of private physicians. The first breakthroughs in the medical profession were cumbersome and awkward formulas for determining whether or not a woman could justify the luxury of deciding what she wanted to do with her reproductive system. These formulas permitted decisions by women who qualified by demonstrating that they suffered from psychiatric disorders, cancer, or critical diseases of one kind or another. Sterilization was first available if clearly necessary for preserving the life or health of the mother. That phrase does sound familiar, doesn't it? It's a reflection of the same attitude and pattern that was so prominent in initial considerations of abortion.

Then the formulas broadened a little and accepted combinations of age versus numbers of children. For example, at any particular hospital a woman who was over forty years of age and had at least three children might not have any problems having her tubes tied. But the woman who was thirty and had only two children might well be refused unless she was willing to endure the humiliation and annoyance of coming up with enough subjective symptoms of excessive menstrual bleeding, pain, discomfort with intercourse, and so forth to convince a sympathetic gynecologist or surgeon to perform a hysterectomy. This was one of the prime reasons there was a great deal of discussion about needless hysterectomies years ago. Women who wanted sterilization were simply given no other direction in which to turn, and medical critics who did not know the truth of the matter cried out in alarm. Many women and their physicians did not have the luxury of simply being able to state that a simpler method of sterilization was the basic need.

Today, honest and straightforward criteria for granting a woman's request for sterilization, regardless of her age, are emerging. There were no problems, for example, in everyone's agreeing to a request such as Noreen's. She was forty-two years old, well preserved in every sense of the word, and enjoyed an active sexual life. Her decision was to end her worries about the bother and minimal risks of contraception for the remaining six, eight, or more years of fertility.

Olga, on the other hand, was thirty-one. She had one child, a thirteen-year-old daughter in school. Her life was happily organized and she had absolutely no interest in wanting to start a family all over again. She didn't quite fit the formulas, but she didn't care. She simply saw no sense in having to worry about contraception for another eighteen to twenty years.

Now consider Prentiss. This bright twenty-six-year-old possessed a degree of maturity and career accomplishment that had already outstripped the achievements of many people much older. She didn't have any children and she never wanted any. Her decision was not a snap judgment and it was not made under stress. She had considered this for years, made a careful decision, and remained committed to her conclusion without second thoughts for a long time. In the course of getting her routine Pap smears and breast checks she had asked at least a half-dozen physicians about a tubal ligation, but the net result had always been the same. Many of them recognized that the average age for considering sterilization had dropped from the forties to the thirties, yet none were prepared to extend that consideration into the twenties, regardless of individual circumstances. The doctors she spoke with were simply unable to place individual needs above the old attitude of the sanctity of fertility. The answers she got tell a revealing story:

"You don't really know what being a woman is all about."

"There is no question that you will meet some nice young man and want to raise a family someday."

"There's no point in seriously discussing this. You're simply too young."

"Now if you had at least two or three children, I wouldn't mind talking with you about it."

"I personally don't care. You look smart enough to know what you want, but there is no way I could pass it through the medical staff."

"Yes, eight years of birth control pills is a long time.

Wouldn't you like to get married or at least try the foams for a while?"

Judging from the sages who refused her, it is obvious why new criteria are coming into existence and why the new criteria will prove stronger and more lasting than the old. Reduced to simple terms, the new criteria include (1) personal maturity, capable of understanding all the implications of a permanent avoidance of pregnancy; (2) a degree of certainty in the decision that indicates there is very little likelihood that even changing future events in a woman's life will alter her decision; and (3) the decision is not being made under pressures of immediate stress. Alternatives must be discussed in this context and snap decisions avoided.

Why are decisions made under stress a bad idea? After an abortion, an unwanted full-term delivery, or following rape, many a teenager has requested sterilization as a form of self-punishment. These women may well reverse their attitudes once immediate pressures fade into the past. On the other hand, women who come to a studied conclusion over several years must be taken seriously. A woman's mature judgment of her own needs must be considered with respect, no matter what her age.

Requests for repairing a tubal ligation are rare. Nevertheless, they are being heard with some increased frequency. Repair can sometimes be accomplished with several techniques, one of which I have published, but no woman should ever be sterilized if she has the slightest idea that she may want to have it changed again at a future time.

Sterilization Procedures for Women. There are only two primary forms of sterilization available. The first involves stopping the functions of a woman's tubes, and the second is hysterectomy, the removal of the uterus. The choice of either of these approaches depends on what each woman needs in terms of her unique physical condition and medical history.

The Fallopian tubes are muscular tubes that transport an egg from an ovary to the uterus. There are many surgical procedures designed to interfere with this function. They include ligation or tying, cutting, coagulating, placement of a permanent band or metal clip around a portion of the tube, or any combination of these things. The net result of all these procedures is about the same, and only very rare failures occur. Most of this small number has been found in ligations that are performed at Caesarean section or following full-term deliveries because of the great blood supply in the pelvis which favors regrowth. A procedure that prevents even these few occurrences is found in the technique I described in the literature several years ago.

A relatively new approach to tubal ligation is called "Band-Aid" surgery. This uses an instrument called a laparoscope, which requires incision so small that it can be covered by only a Band-Aid. It offers the advantages of a very short hospital stay, almost unnoticeable cosmetic effects, rapid recovery, instant protection, and lower cost than most other procedures. The efficiency of reliability of this technique is approximately one thousand to one.

"What happens to all the eggs?" is a frequently asked question. The answer is simple. Any egg that is not fertilized disintegrates within a matter of days.

"How will this affect my sex life or my periods?" is another common question. The answer to this one is also straightforward. The primary function of the tubes is to transport an egg. When that function is eliminated pregnancy cannot occur because there will be no meeting of the egg with sperm. Nothing else is changed because nothing else is involved.

The removal of the uterus, known as a hysterectomy, is a larger surgical procedure than a tubal ligation. It is more costly, involves more time in the hospital, and requires a longer recovery. It does have a place in the consideration of sterilization because a hysterectomy may provide other medical benefits, depending on a woman's physical condition. For example, the woman who has fibroid tumors causing specific problems on her uterus, or other conditions resulting in excessive bleeding, severe pain, discomfort with intercourse, loss of bladder control, and a host of other conditions, may have these problems corrected surgically, with sterilization a welcome secondary benefit. Since about one out of every twenty-five women is likely to develop a form of uterine cancer, this potential problem is eliminated also. Once again, this decision is a matter of consultation between a woman and her physician.

One point about hysterectomy needs to be made over and over again. Most people have incredibly inaccurate ideas of what a hysterectomy is, which is no more than removing the uterus. *It has no effect on the ovaries or any other part of a woman's anatomy.*

Exactly what is the uterus and what does it do? It is simply a hollow muscle, and its only function is to grow babies. If it does not receive a fertilized egg by the end of each menstrual cycle, its lining sheds and it bleeds. That's all there is to it. The uterus has no effect on a woman's ovaries, which produce her female sexual hormones. Contrary to the mythology of the past several thousand years, there is absolutely no "cleansing effect" during the process of menstruation. Other than being the shedding of the lining of the uterus that prepared for a pregnancy every month, menstruation has absolutely no value to anyone but shareholders in pad and tampon manufacturing companies.

A hysterectomy brings about only three things: the elimination of pregnancy, the elimination of menstrual bleeding, and the elimination of any problems referable to the uterus itself. There are no other physical, emotional, chemical, sexual, hormonal, or other changes of any kind.

Last but not least, elimination of menstrual periods does not mean placement into the menopause. The menopause begins when the ovaries no longer produce eggs and no longer produce the hormonal changes required for completing a full menstrual cycle. This process occurs in its own good time with or without the presence of a uterus.

A hysterectomy is not the recommended cure for the desire not to have an additional pregnancy, but may be of great help when specific problems over and above the need for sterilization do exist.

Sterilization for Men. A vasectomy is the male equivalent of a tubal ligation. It is a fairly simple and rapid procedure in which the duct that carries sperm from the testicles to the penis is tied and separated. This is usually done under a local anesthetic in a physician's office.

What does a vasectomy do to a man? There is no interference with any aspect of masculinity, interest in sex, or quality of performance. There is normal ejaculation of a normal amount of fluid with every orgasm. If anything, most men respond with an increased sexual interest because they realize that they no longer have to worry about impregnating a partner.

The most common reason for a vasectomy is a couple's decision to avoid future children. Most of the time, they choose vasectomy because it is the least involved and least expensive sterilization technique.

The next most common reason reflects "men's liberation" from fatherhood. Some men want to enjoy *their* sexual rights with no pregnancy worries. These men generally have a strong feeling of being considerate and fair to the one or more loves in their lives. They seem to have the attitude encapsulated in the slogan "Shoot blanks and fire often," and many women enjoy the security of these partners.

There are a few words of caution that must be mentioned about this procedure. The first is that the effectiveness of a vasectomy is good but not foolproof. On rare occasions the ducts grow back together. When this happens and the man's partner becomes pregnant there is an inevitable discussion about the source of the pregnancy. To prevent the serious accusations that are sometimes leveled against this woman, a man with a vasectomy should have his sperm count checked every couple of years. Overall, a tubal ligation is considered more reliable than a vasectomy.

The second note of caution reflects a dirty trick that sends a small but unforgettable number of women to my clinic. There is the sick, rare man who deceives a woman into believing that he has had a vasectomy when he is all too fertile. Unfortunately, women have little defense against this demented type of man other than to be aware of his existence. I would estimate that approximately one out of five hundred unwanted pregnancies is attributable to this cause. The real incidence could be higher.

Finally, there are some men who should not have a vasectomy, just as there are women who should not have a tubal ligation or hysterectomy. Snap decisions for sterilization and judgments made under pressure are no better for men than they are for women. Men have less difficulty in arranging to have a sterilizing procedure performed than women, but by the same token they may have less counseling and review of their thinking on this decision.

Adequate review is necessary for a vasectomy, just as it is required in any surgical procedure. For example, there are a small number of men who have a deep-seated equation of masculinity with fertility, just as some women equate fertility with the fulfillment of their role in life. It's important to recognize that men also have emotions and needs that must be considered in good conscience before a vasectomy is performed.

8

RESOLVING FEELINGS FROM AN ABORTION IN THE PAST

Occasionally, some of the mothers or fathers who bring their daughters to the clinic want to talk about their own past problems. One woman in particular stands out above many others in my memory because what she had to say covered so many things mentioned in so many similar stories. My secretary buzzed me between procedures one day and asked if I would talk with one of the mothers whose sixteen-year-old daughter was having a procedure.

"I came hoping for the best for Arlene," she said. "I'm happy to be able to say we've found it. I wanted to thank you personally and, well, to tell you things have come a long way since I was young. You see, I had to have an abortion myself back then. It's a shame you weren't here twenty-five years ago. Things were a lot different. An illegal abortion was really a bad situation."

Rachel was a handsome gray-haired woman in her early fifties who had a pleasant mixture of warmth and concern. She wanted to talk about one of the most important experiences in her life, one that was bottled up for many, many years. "You know, Arlene was scared today until we spoke with your counselor. I understand that feeling very, very well. It's a shame that she has to go through it at all. But at least she is safe and *can* talk about it. At least she can be treated like a human being."

"What happened?" I asked.

She looked up at the ceiling for a moment, then began. "Times were pretty bad and I had a child already. I was only twenty-three at the time. My husband decided that he was just tired of it all. He wasn't angry or anything. He just gave up. He started staying away from home, spending more and more time with other people and other women, I'm sure. Once he disappeared for three weeks at a time. He said that he was looking for new work. Finally, he left for good. He sent a note which simply said: 'I won't be back.'

"In the meantime I found out that I was pregnant. I was so upset that I couldn't eat. Once I took a half bottle of sleeping pills but it just made me sick. I threw up for days. I didn't know where to turn. My parents found out and they wanted to help. There was no real choice. But I couldn't talk much to them then. They made some arrangement. My father drove me all the way to New Mexico. We arrived in town in the late afternoon and had to hang around until nighttime. Somebody met us and took us out to a fairly elaborate set of offices that looked like an old Spanish mansion from the movies. I still remember a big grandfather clock that scared me. It's silly the things you remember.

"At least this place looked okay. I was really afraid of winding up in a barn or on the floor of some vacant apartment. I knew about a lot of girls who did exactly that. They had to go through with it and it was really horrible. They told about no medication, nobody to talk to, just a shot of whiskey and a cloth to chew in your mouth while some people held your shoulders down and your legs apart. It was just horrible, the things they said. I heard about the coat hangers and things shoved inside. I knew that many of them got sick and some even died.

"I guess it must have cost a lot. I was scared out of my wits but things weren't as bad as the stories I'd heard. The worst thing was that no one talked to me. I felt like some criminal that was just going to be executed one way or another, and should be grateful if it could be done without hurting too much. A big woman there looked sympathetic, but she wouldn't answer any questions. I guess I panicked. It was bad. I remember being picked up bodily and fighting some man who held a mask over my face. It must have been ether. It made me violently sick and throw up on the floor. It did work, though, because I don't remember any pain, just bad cramps and a lot of bleeding when I came to. My father was upset about all the bleeding but the doctor ... I think he was a doctor ... didn't want us hanging around town because of publicity. We had to leave and didn't even know if we could tell my doctor back home. All in all, I guess I was lucky. It could have been worse."

"How do you feel about it today?" I asked.

"I've thought about it ever since then, and have never been happy about it. I'm more sorry that it had to happen than that it did. But that's easier to say now. Back then I knew there was no choice, but I could never say what I felt to anybody, not even to my parents. I think that's what made me go through so many years of feeling guilty and ashamed. Not even one person ever said, 'I understand.'

"I didn't want things to work out that way and I wanted a husband and family ... all the things you're supposed to enjoy. Sometimes I stop and wonder what things might have been like if my first marriage had worked out, because I have nothing but an empty feeling from it. One part of me says that everything worked out for the best. It really has, you know, but another part won't let me forget that emptiness."

"What have been your biggest problems?" I asked.

"All these years, I haven't been sure how everybody would look at me if they knew what I had done. When I was growing up, having babies was supposed to be good and everything else was bad. Until last week I never told anyone but my second husband what happened, and I didn't tell him until we'd been married ten years. I wanted to talk to someone, desperately, but there wasn't anyone I dared tell. At first, I wanted someone to tell me how to react and feel, even though it happened to me. I just didn't know how to think about myself. I didn't want anyone to say that it was good or bad, I just wanted someone to stand back and help me see it the way it was.

"The first couple of years were hard." She sighed. "I stayed away from people. My mother thought I might even be going over the edge. But because I was skittish, nobody bothered me much. Most people figured I was upset because my husband had taken off, and of course that was true. The funny thing about it was that I had stopped caring about him or anyone. On my part, I felt that if I just took care of my son, that would fill the gap and make up for all the rest of it."

"Were you happy with that?" I asked.

"I was never happy back then, but I got over it. It took a long time and I figured out something that helped. Life doesn't work by substitutions. Being busy with my son was fine, but it didn't make up for the one I didn't have. You see, when I came home from the hospital after being pregnant there were rough times, too, but there was something to show for it, which was a baby I could feel good about. The problem after New Mexico was that there wasn't anything to show for it other than doing something to heal a bad wound. To this day I'm not sure how much of that wound resulted from the abortion and how much was caused by the problems before and after it. The emptiness filled slowly, like the way things fill in after a tooth is pulled—it hurts a lot, something is missing, but after a while things can work again."

My sympathies were aroused. As a young woman, Rachel's abortion had thoroughly disoriented her, but in front of me was a well-adjusted, middle-aged mother. I asked her to explain how she had got over her sorrows.

"That part took much longer. For a while I tried to be a working mother and faithful daughter. Trying to shut out the rest of the world wasn't enough, because it made my life a stagnant routine. It had no interest, no vitality, no enrichment, there was no way I felt I was growing. I used to get very upset about this. I realized that I was sort of working off a debt that I had to pay, even though I didn't ask for that debt to begin with. But like I said, you can't substitute past a certain point, and when I saw this, I felt better and started dating again, or at least getting out of the house.

"That was another thing. The whole idea of sex absolutely vanished. It just disappeared. I would never have believed that you could get so thoroughly turned off on this. That frightened me. I thought I had been so upset about this whole experience that I would never think like a normal woman, never feel like a woman, or act like a woman again. There was no point in talking about it to anyone. I wouldn't actually ask anybody what they thought, but I tried to joke about it or mention it in passing. I hoped that somebody would say something very clever, profound, maybe even helpful. They either thought it was funny, would not take it seriously, or just passed the whole thing off with one remark or another.

"And now I'll tell you something even stranger. When I started feeling like I wanted to be with a man again, it scared me even more. I was really worried to the point where I finally did go to my doctor. That was a useless waste of time. The best he could come up with was that I was probably still in love with my husband. I didn't think that was the answer, and I got together the courage to go see a psychiatrist."

"What did the psychiatrist say?" I asked. I was interested in hearing the advice she was given twenty years ago.

"I was surprised. He said something that really helped. Frankly, I only expected a bunch of mumbo-jumbo. He said not to worry, and he gave me a reason that turned out to be true. Things come, but only in their time. Things happen when they are ready and you can't turn them on or off that easily in any other way. He told me that when I was ready to have a new relationship, to love someone again, to whatever, I would know and I would act accordingly. Trying to worry into it or out of it, to speed it up or slow it down or even getting aggravated about it was foolish because time would heal me. I didn't have to worry about bending myself out of shape or trying to fit into it one way or another.

"He talked about the word *comfortable*. I'll never forget that as long as I live. He said, 'All the things you were raised with, all the things that feel good and hurt, come down to that one word. You could take a week, and a dozen people helping you to get to a single decision you have to make, but it is a lot quicker and better to think about whether you are comfortable doing something or not. Comfortable doesn't always mean happy in rough decisions. You were certainly not happy about having an abortion and all the things that led up to it, but you had to feel comfortable in your decision and the lives of your parents and child. It is the same thing with being ready to get back among the living with sex, socializing, or whatever. When you are ready for a relationship you will be comfortable with it, and you will act accordingly.' "

Rachel paused as if she had just recalled all that advice for the first time in some years, and was feeling afresh the impact it had on her. "It's so different for Arlene... and I'm so glad that she won't have to go through the needless hell that I did.

"When I found out that she was pregnant and couldn't keep it, I was shocked. I can't tell you how much. It brought everything back to me, and for a moment it seemed like I was being punished again for the problems I had so many years ago, whether I deserved them or not. I went through the hell of reliving a curse. And then I realized that everyone has her own problems and one generation does not pass on immunity to another. I couldn't stop thinking about what I had been through and it hurt badly all over again. And I thought of how it could have been different, better, easier for me... and now I was scared for my daughter. What worried me most was... did I have the wisdom to handle myself and help her, too?

"When she told us she was pregnant, Arlene was scared. I talked to my husband and we decided to talk to her about what happened to me. Would you believe that Arlene wound up comforting me? It was unreal. It was the weirdest mixture of emotions I've ever had or ever expect to feel again.

"Today, your counselor helped so very much. I listened to everything she spoke about and heard it for myself as well. The questions she brought up! Did Arlene consider all the possibilities? Did she think about how her decision would affect her life and everyone else in it? Did she feel secure that abortion *was* her best choice? What reached me most was, how did she think it might affect her life later. These are scary things to go into, but they are beautiful, because they do have answers and those answers come up front. They don't have to hurt through wasted years of doubt and agony.

"You know, I felt like a real idiot while all this talking was going on. Arlene had things together. I almost envied her and I was proud of her strength. I was the one who was crying. Some was for the pain she was going through. Some, or maybe most, was for the realization that her pain would be less than mine."

"Rachel, your daughter knows you understand," I said. "You have become the person you were looking for twenty-five years ago, the person who should have said, 'I understand.' Now, your strength is helping your daughter. You needed it then. As things turned out, she needs you now. She's grateful, just as you would have been back then. You haven't given her release from her problem. It is hers, and always will be. You have given her relief from excessive, needless pain. And that is a gift which, I am sure, has made so much of your own suffering worthwhile."

III

NEW FINDINGS: A FOUR-YEAR SUMMARY

To this point, you have seen the realities of unexpected pregnancy as it exists today. Now the time has come to bring you into the big picture of its underlying causes and patterns. This is no longer a curious problem affecting only other people. It is one aspect of the many changes taking place today in women's responses to themselves, their children, husbands, and lovers.

9

HIDDEN CAUSES OF MILLIONS OF UNWANTED PREGNANCIES

The Great Maternity Trap

Despite decades of scientific research, today's most commonly used contraceptive is *the intention to abstain from sex*. Literally thousands of women have wound up at my clinic because they had not planned on having intercourse. They thought they didn't need birth control, then found themselves unprotected when they had sex.

Consider Florence, a young woman who was engaged but planned to avoid intercourse until marriage. She didn't use birth control because she didn't plan to have sex. In other words, she intended to use abstinence to prevent pregnancy. It didn't work.

Patty, for example, was thirty and recently divorced. She dated often but felt she knew enough to avoid sex until she had a single relationship, at which time she would definitely use birth control. Being without companionship was harder than she expected. Sex began soon —without contraceptives.

Then there was Inez, who had a different attitude. She was twenty-four and had never married. She didn't have the slightest interest in contraception because, as she explained it, "No man will touch me before I'm good and ready." When she met her Mr. Right all her other emotions were more absorbing than the worry about birth control.

Nanci, on the other hand, had a husband who had a vasectomy. She thought she had no reason to protect herself, and she never intended to have more than a friendship outside her marriage. After several years her resolution disappeared in the reality of an affair.

All these women, and countless others like them, intended to abstain from intercourse. They wound up at an abortion clinic instead. The intention of abstinence is a pitfall because this intention, to put it bluntly, may well be unrealistic.

Nature, evolution, and God have made sex an unavoidable and extremely rewarding need. It is true that this biological drive is at odds with society's training to suppress many kinds of sexual interest and expression. But as a gynecologist with eighteen years of practice, and as the medical director of a busy clinic for women, I must put all my experience behind this fact: I have seen instinctive programing almost always win over the social desire to restrain sex to narrow limits, given enough chance and time.

The truth of the matter is that sex is more than part of who we are. It is part of *what* we are. The urge to sexual activity is instinctive, strong, and undeniable. Caring for a person so much that it leads to a sexual experience is a social response. Both the caring and that urge may become inseparable. They can be contained, modified, and even suppressed. But they are too powerful a combination for most people to disregard for very long. *Sex is a biological fact that is beyond social licensure.*

The social command to refrain from "unlicensed"

sex is a general guide that most people do follow most of the time. It offers a false security as a reliable form of birth control. An instinctive call to sexual activity exists, and it cannot always be denied by even the most severe social training. If a woman has *enjoyed* sex once, the intention to abstain from sex may have validity but may not be dependable in all situations and at all times.

A new conclusion has emerged from our experience at the clinic, and like so many of our other findings, it is powerful: *Every fertile woman who has enjoyed sexual contact must be considered a candidate for birth control, even if she has every intention of abstaining from intercourse.*

Am I saying that *every* woman who may need it should have immediately available some form of contraceptive? I most certainly am. The time for an unrealistic, "nice philosophy of life" is past. If the number of unwanted pregnancies is to be reduced, contraceptives must be used.

It's inevitable. This concept may not be accepted gracefully by some people. Their argument is simple: "If my daughter goes on the pill, it will be a license for her to have sex." This argument seems to make sense, but it demonstrates three serious defects. First, the idea of sexual intercourse is not taken lightly by most women, whether they use birth control or not. Second, interest in sexual activity is a biological drive that is beyond licensure. Once a woman has enjoyed sex she has been granted her own instinctive authority. Third, the woman who uses contraception certainly has a choice of sexual decision. *Contraception protects her without invalidating her choice.*

The alternative is pressure to keep women away from contraceptives. This puts them into a dangerous trap. It implies that a woman without protection will not have intercourse, and this is a false premise.

Parents who put their philosophy above the safety of their daughters will reject these uncomfortable facts in disgust. Those who have a sincere concern for their daughter's safety will consider them well.

The attempt to avoid sex altogether is only the first kind of abstinence. "It's okay to play around as long as we don't go all the way," is a second way to attempt abstinence. If that phrase sounds even slightly familiar, it is easy to appreciate how common it is. Many teenage and some adult couples use this attitude to share themselves and enjoy various kinds of orgasms, but stop before intercourse. As a method of contraception for any duration, it is a noble gesture doomed to failure.

In a third kind of abstinence, a little bit of insertion is not a little bit of intercourse. Coitus interruptus (withdrawal or pulling out) is not reliable. Sperm appears in the seminal fluid long before ejaculation. Even if both partners do separate while all their emotional and physical needs urge them to stay joined, there is a good chance that they are too late. A little bit of insertion can lead to a whole lot of pregnancy.

Couples who are interested in planning their family realistically should also recognize the limits of another variation of abstinence, the rhythm system. A small but surprising number of women express shock at becoming pregnant when they use it since, they say, "I had intercourse only in the middle of the month and never before or after menstruation." Believe it or not, this really does happen.

The rhythm system is based on the assumption that an average woman with average fertility having an average menstrual cycle will be fertile on the average on day twelve to fourteen after the onset of her menstrual period. The good news is that these *averages* are true. The bad news is that there is no guarantee that next month's ovulation will occur on the same day as in previous months. From time to time ovaries adopt a different rhythm of their own. Most women who use the rhythm system sooner or later say, "But it worked for years!" These averages are useful for explaining a simplified picture of how ovulation usually works, but the woman who has an unwanted pregnancy is one hundred percent pregnant.

In my opinion the rhythm system is a fine way for couples to play at family spacing. If a woman cannot cope with another pregnancy, however, she must recognize this approach as a thinly veiled maternity trap. The periodic abstinence known as the rhythm system may prevent pregnancy—or it may only delay it.

An interesting variation of abstinence is its opposite, superfrequent sex. Some people know of the medical advice given to couples who are having difficulty conceiving a child. These couples are told to wait forty-eight hours between occasions of intercourse because it takes that long for a male to build a full sperm count. From this information some people conclude that daily intercourse or masturbation before intercourse will prevent pregnancy. This conclusion can lead to pregnancy very quickly.

In the end, it turns out that the intention to abstain from sex is more frequent than most people think. It is an overwhelming realization that this intention is one of the most relied on forms of birth control today—and the most unreliable.

Our society will not be able to reduce its large number of unwanted pregnancies until it recognizes that the intent to abstain from sex fails in practice, that every fertile woman who has enjoyed sex must use birth control or have it immediately available. Unless this advice is followed, any woman who is not on contraceptives runs the constant risk of becoming pregnant.

In addition to women who plan to abstain from sex,

many sexually active women who do not want to become pregnant reject contraceptives. This refusal has nothing to do with religious faith. It is an unjustified equation of contraception with promiscuity.

The Promiscuity-contraception Connection

This second largest cause of unwanted pregnancy is one of my clinic's most significant discoveries. It has little to do with a lack of knowledge, a lack of funds, or promiscuity, as is generally supposed. Many sexually active women simply do not use birth control, even though they do not want to become pregnant. We have investigated why this occurs with such astonishing frequency, and have found in these women a nearly universal negative association of promiscuity with contraception, instilled by society in many subtle ways, and reinforced from childhood on.

The Denial of Sexual Reality. It sounds normal and proper that many teenage women should tell us, "I would never ask my parents for birth control pills, because they would just about kill me." These young women know that if they ask for contraceptives, their parents will assume it is because they need to use them. If a young woman needs to use birth control, parents conclude that she's having a sexual relationship she probably shouldn't have.

These teenage women are saying that they have already absorbed the connection between contraception and promiscuity. They may have learned it directly, if their parents said, "I don't want you to be *that* kind of girl," or, "You know you're not supposed to be fooling around with boys." It might have been taught to them indirectly, with even greater strength, when their parents spoke about the girls in school who got caught in sexual affairs, and,

"Aren't they really tramps? I hope you never do anything like that."

These direct and indirect messages hit most young women hard. They not only feel inhibited from asking for contraception if they need it, but they are also imprinted with a negative association that lasts for years, in most cases throughout their entire lives: "If I use contraception I'm *that* kind of woman."

By her late teenage years a woman reaches physical maturity and possesses some authority in running her own life. She doesn't have to ask her parents' permission for contraceptives, but she still has to ask a physician or a pharmacist, with or without her parents' knowledge. The attitudes of many physicians contribute to making a young patient reluctant to request birth control. Many of these young women have told me that they decided to try contraceptive foam, but felt awkward and embarrassed when they went to pay for it. Logically, a woman should know that a pharmacist or drugstore clerk couldn't care less whether she is married, single, or divorced.

The next step in a woman's development is critical. It occurs in her early twenties, when she has used her own judgment enough to lose many worries about what other people think. By this time a woman is supposedly free to form her own opinions, and some women do realize that contraception is a necessary part of nearly every sexual encounter. At this time the previous judgments have been burned deeply enough into most women's attitudes to be translated into their opinion of themselves.

Bernadette, for example, was born in 1942. Since she grew up with World War II values, she never had the occasion to ask for or need contraception until she was a full twenty-one years of age. Whenever sex was mentioned in her family, it was implied that it is something unclean that other people did. She used to laugh at this stuffy attitude and mischievously wonder how she was conceived at all. Despite this hint of reality, she was comfortable keeping herself "straight."

In college, however, Bernadette met a young man whose company she liked and who made her feel very deeply the real stimulation she had only heard her girlfriends talk about previously. Neither of them visualized getting married, and much to her own surprise she wasn't even sure she wanted to get married. Contraception was an easy answer, but Bernadette never considered it seriously. She did get pregnant, and since this was the early 1960s, she had an illegal abortion. It was her only alternative.

We saw Bernadette shortly after the clinic opened. She was thirty and hadn't married, partly because of the trauma she suffered from her first abortion. When we talked to her, we saw a well-educated, somewhat attractive woman who was clearly in command of her life. She had had a total of three relationships, the second of which lasted many years. Although there was moderately frequent intercourse in all her relationships, this woman's image of herself would never allow her to admit that she had ever had an affair. Even the suggestion that she might have been promiscuous would horrify her.

To Bernadette, obtaining birth control pills, an IUD, diaphragm, or whatever, and using them faithfully would be a confession that sex was an important part of her life. That, in her opinion, would certainly classify her as a promiscuous woman.

In point of fact, Bernadette had never been promiscuous. She never even took the trouble to find out what this really is. She knew that "promiscuous" is an easy label to pin on someone, and that it's bad. She didn't realize that its meaning is closer to the word *casual* than to the word *often*. Bernadette was incapable of a casual relationship. Although she had slept with three men in her life, by no means could she be called a promiscuous woman.

In her discussion with the counselor, Bernadette revealed that she hated the idea of a second abortion, but she felt desperate and couldn't do anything else. She said she was in the same situation as when she'd had her first abortion. Neither she nor her boyfriend was ready to get married. It turned out that even though this third relationship had already lasted a year and a half, she hadn't talked about the pregnancy with her boyfriend. My counselor suggested that she think about her decision more, and talk to her boyfriend extensively. Bernadette called a week later to tell the counselor that after an evening's deep talk about everything inside them, he had opened up and said, "You know, I'm really glad. Deep down inside, I've been thinking about marriage. I really don't want you to have an abortion."

Bernadette grew up with the attitude that she would never be "that" kind of woman. During her twenties she knew the shock of an unwanted pregnancy, but rejected birth control because she felt she had a "deeper understanding of life," and "would be very careful." Of course, there isn't any way to be "careful" that works. Her attitude represented a subconscious inhibition instead of a realistic alternative.

These attitudes about contraception also have a powerful influence on divorced women who married when they were young, used birth control "with a clear conscience" during their marriage—even for ten or fifteen years—but then became single again. A divorced woman is just as apt to resist contraception in her twenties, thirties, and forties as she did in her teenage years, and for the same reasons.

The idea of going out on a date "fully prepared for

action" is repulsive to many divorced women. This denial of a very real sexual potential is exactly why this woman is likely to have an unwanted pregnancy at any time, right up to the distant end of her fertile life. "Doc, I never thought I'd meet someone this soon," or, "I never dreamed we'd go to bed together on the first or second date," are comments I often hear from pregnant women who are divorced.

Completing the circle, women who connect contraceptives with promiscuity are likely to do everything in their power to transmit their attitude to their daughters. Many mothers of teenage women have said, "If I had the pill when I was my kid's age, even I might have gotten into trouble. You can be sure I'm not going to let her have the pill." Their daughters have taken their mothers' attitudes to heart. An unforgettable number of teenage women who have an abortion reject contraceptives because of their upbringing—despite the fact that they are likely to remain sexually active. They have the misguided impression that using contraceptives makes them a "tramp," even though the relationships within which they are sexually active are deeply felt and sincere. Without protection, these young women could easily encounter another unwanted pregnancy.

Why a High Percentage of Catholics? Bernadette did not happen to be Catholic. Her training was strong, but did not specifically condemn birth control. Young Catholic women not only have to contend with a negative reaction to birth control from their parents and within themselves, they also have to contend with their image before God.

This explains a finding that seemed totally unbelievable when we started compiling our first statistics soon after the clinic opened. The same statistical pattern has continued to the present day. Overall, 38 percent of the women requesting abortion in our area are Catholic, while the general population in the area is approximately 22 percent Catholic.

This pattern offers substantial support for the promiscuity-contraception connection. Certainly, the Catholic women in the area are no more promiscuous than non-Catholics, and they are at least as religious. The conflict between birth control and abortion has proven absolutely overwhelming to many Catholic women. On one side is the ill-fated rhythm system and the prohibition against birth control, which sooner or later may lead to an unwanted pregnancy. Most Catholic women know this and feel it is unacceptable. The bottom line is not wanting endless pregnancies, but at the same time not wanting to walk around with a constant feeling of guilt.

All women are heir to the problem of pregnancy, regardless of their religious backgrounds. Simplistic answers such as, "Behave yourself and you won't need contraception or abortion," don't hold water. Those who are able to feel for the problems of others, over and above their upbringing, have voiced their feelings in the many public opinion polls that show that the majority of Catholics favor the continued availability of safe, legal abortion.

Maria was a traditional Catholic. The conflict she faced in her fifth pregnancy horrified her. Even though this pregnancy wasn't a medical threat to her life, she decided to have an abortion because she felt it was her only realistic answer. She was very upset, and knew many people who would condemn her if they found out what she did. Some might say her emotional scars from the experience serve her right, some might have more compassion.

As you might suspect, and in the face of the terrible time she went through, Maria could not bring herself to accept birth control after the abortion. Those without compassion shouldn't feel satisfied, because this crisis could easily overwhelm her again. A threatening cloud hangs over all her intimate thinking for the rest of her fertile years.

The Two-week Sweats: A Traumatic Absolution. The menstrual cycle forces women who don't use contraceptives to suffer a major trauma every month. Louise was a married woman in her early thirties, a Southern Baptist, and worked for the same man for about six years as a well-paid executive secretary. They were close friends, though not lovers. Gradually, she took the place of his wife, after his wife disappeared one day, leaving him two young daughters, about three years after Louise had been working for him.

Their friendship benefited them both. "I never thought we would become sexually involved," she said. "I knew that it could happen, but neither of us wanted to start an affair. We didn't want to upset the wonderful ways we worked and talked together.

"After about five years the eventual happened," she said. "And it seemed right and natural and almost even proper ... except it wasn't proper and we both knew it was wrong. I feel like a fool now, but I didn't want to use birth control because that would make our beautiful relationship into something bad. And every time I got a period, would you believe it, it felt like a sign that everything was all right. I know that sounds crazy, but it's true.

"You'd think I'd be smart enough to know better. Time after time, waiting for my period turned into a horrible ordeal. I was forced to think about the effects on his family, and had the chilling realization that if I became pregnant I could become unwelcome in his life forever. That's what hurt the most. I know the answer should have been simple: 'Be smart, use the pill or something. Forget all the nonsense about proving a point for love and beauty.' But I just couldn't give in to it and go on the pill. Foolish as it was, I needed the feeling that something special and wonderful, something more than just taking a pill for sex, was a real part of my life.

"About six months ago we started having sex often and worrying about it all the time. And then every time I had my period we both felt like we had a fresh start again. Two months ago everything went wrong, because I got pregnant. I couldn't believe that something that always turned out right could be destroyed for no really good reason."

Louise was not very realistic. She was raised to think in terms of black and white, and this background led her straight to an unwanted pregnancy. In her case, as in so many others, her feelings about what is right for her, and her conditioning about birth control, did not come out together in a neat, gratifying answer. She grasped the only way she could live with herself at the time. "How is it possible," she asked, "that something can be right and good and wrong all at the same time?"

The promiscuity-contraception delusion is an amazingly common attitude that is found in all kinds of relationships. People will respond to their emotions sexually, but "If I use birth control I'll have to think of myself as loose" is an almost frightening viewpoint, because it causes hundreds of thousands of unexpected pregnancies every year. It is right that women should enjoy their sexuality, but it is a mistake when they feel that intercourse is made shameful by the use of birth control.

Sex within a meaningful relationship is a central part of almost everyone's life. A woman who sincerely cares for a man does not have to think of herself as wild or loose if she uses birth control. Contraception is an admission that a woman is sexually active, or simply has a sexual potential, but this does not mean promiscuous. It should mean healthy, normal, and happy. Besides, birth control removes the end-of-every-month trauma of possible pregnancy that can explode suddenly into the crisis of an abortion.

The Sexual Adulthood of Teenage Women

Difficult New Demands on Parents. When a thirteen-year-old female becomes pregnant, she isn't anything less than an adult woman. This kind of adulthood is often shocking to the young woman's parents, yet it is strikingly common. Nearly one out of five women who has an abortion at my clinic is under the age of eighteen.

These women's adolescence—the years when they are under the emotional guidance of their parents—has shortened considerably since their parents were teenagers. Today, society encourages children to mature rapidly, and parents do too. But when parents expect their daughters to remain sexually naïve while they grow up quickly, serious family problems are the typical result.

Michelle's pregnancy exemplifies this all too common pattern. She was a fifteen-year-old blonde who wore a childlike purple dress that barely contained a body developed far beyond her years. On the morning I saw her she was misty-eyed because she didn't want to upset her parents or anyone else. She had found a warm relationship with a young man graduating high school, and this made up for the closeness she rarely received at home.

Michelle's parents wanted to see me rather than a counselor, and I noticed her father first. He remained standing after everyone had sat down, and dominated the discussion.

"I told her she was too young to start going out. Where does a fifteen-year-old get off messing around?" He began pacing the office. "I could understand if she were some freaky hippie kid who hung out with motorcycle gangs, or if we didn't care about her. But she does come from a good home. Then she pulls this stunt. I'd be ready to let her have a baby and find out what life is about, but I'd have to take care of it."

Daddy's face was red at this point, and the veins stood out on his head and neck. It seemed that he was more interested in beating himself in public for having failed as a "father" than in sharing his feelings with his wife and daughter.

Michelle was lost somewhere between helpless and hopeless. She looked to her mother for help. Her mother answered by pursing her lips and lowering her eyes to the floor. It was a safe bet that this approach for help had been denied many times, right through the moment when Michelle wanted to ask for birth control pills.

Why had Michelle's mother let her daughter down? It probably came from the ground rules of what is proper behavior for a "good mother," as laid down by Big Daddy. Now she just had one last chance to take Michelle's outstretched hand in her own, and she blew it. It was obvious that this woman felt guilty, and the questions that seemed to haunt her were, "How am I going to talk with Michelle again? I really love her. I guess she's not a little girl after all. How can I be her friend?"

It's sad how so much unhappiness began with something very nice and almost beautiful. Michelle herself said, when we were alone, she really didn't want to do anything bad, just be close to this young man. She knew that women her age could become pregnant. It had happened to several of her friends and there was hell to pay for it. But she knew that if she asked for birth control pills, just like that, her father would flat out kill her and that would be the end of it.

For Michelle, the window of sincere communication

between her and her parents was closed by her pregnancy. Her parents hadn't looked at her directly for days, except in anger. She was frightened, upset, and confused. I had to reassure her that she wasn't a rotten person just because her parents were unhappy with her.

Michelle wanted an abortion because it would end the whole thing. The way she looked when her father was carrying on and her mother had emotionally abandoned her was that she wanted to die quietly, and would have been grateful if she could have done so.

The Closing Window of Time. Many parents who grew up with World War II values of black and white, right and wrong, cannot do as much as they would like to supervise a teenager's orientation into adult life today. The values that shaped their own more slowly developing maturity no longer apply to the teenage years of their children, particularly their daughters. The result is a large group of parents with a deep and upsetting sense of panic.

Various books and discussions have called this change the new morality. Most of these have not helped because they do not define the basic difference between the extended adolescence parents experienced and the accelerated maturity of their children. Repeated family confrontations with reality, on a daily basis in the clinic, have made a new definition and solution clear.

The most helpful picture of adolescence is to see it as a "window of time" during which meaningful emotional guidelines for coping with adulthood are transmitted from parent to child. In the clinic we have observed that this window has shrunk almost to the point of closing, though it has not disappeared.

Why is this window of time closing? The parents' side closes because they see their daughters as children who have already developed shockingly different values

from what they knew. Parents try to offer guidance, sometimes forcefully, in an attempt to control their child's
behavior. The less they respect their daughter's self-made
choices the sooner they compel her to declare her emotional independence. Then, when the young woman ma-
tures sexually on her own in spite of her parents' disap-
proval, she often is deemed rebellious.

The young woman's side closes because society encourages her sexual awareness at an early age. The pregnant young women we see at the clinic are usually bright,
perceptive, sincere, and warm people—adults in every
sense of the word except for their age and their parents'
opinions. Most of them enjoy the idea of growing up and
learning about the world for themselves.

Some parents do understand and support their daughters. When a young woman's self-direction is accomplished
gracefully and with the approval of her parents it is called
early maturation. For today's generation of teenagers, this
is normal.

One point must be understood by parents: *The parent should not interpret their child's sexual independence
as a personal, parental failure.* This sense of failure is the
common, emotionally upsetting reaction most parents
bring to the clinic. It intensifies a family's existing problems far beyond an unwanted pregnancy. If this difference
in values is pressed too hard, it can produce a complete
emotional break between a young woman and her parents.

This is both unnecessary and tragic. Most modern
parents are neither inadequate nor have they failed in
their attempt to prepare their children for a realistic entrance into adulthood. On the contrary, these problems
arise because parents have *succeeded* in helping their children mature faster than they did. The answer for parents
lies in the realization that they must begin both emotional
and rational communication at the earliest time their child

can absorb it, usually by the time they are *young* teenagers *who see themselves as adults and expect to be treated as adults.*

Family communications are sometimes revealed at the clinic in a dramatic way. Jody was a self-possessed, tall and mature-looking sixteen-year-old woman. Her parents, boyfriend, and minister accompanied her to the clinic. It didn't take long to realize that all of these people had a deep love and respect for one another. I remember her well because my initial reaction was to question why these people were considering terminating a pregnancy. Something was wrong.

That something turned out to be quite overwhelming. Jody described her situation herself. "I should have never let this happen, because I can't keep the pregnancy. About six months ago my doctor found that I have a malignancy and I may only have a couple of years to live. Even if I do make out all right, I don't know what all the medicine and stuff will do to the pregnancy." She looked down at her hands which were folded in her lap. "I should have never let this happen, because now there is no good way out."

Jody's parents, boyfriend, and minister were looking at her, feeling every word. Her mother encouraged her to go on. "We all talked about it a lot. I knew what was going on and I feel stupid because I knew what to do for birth control." She paused, then continued in a softer voice. "I had to make the decision myself and I think it's all right because it's not that I don't want to have a baby and it's not even so much that it wouldn't be taken care of. My parents said that I shouldn't worry and that if I wanted to have it they'd take care of it. That's really fantastic. They're really great. But I don't think that would be right, even if I could help . . . I mean even if my health was okay."

At this point she didn't have the strength to keep going. Everyone spoke and expressed deep, sincere feelings, but the minister who was with her best summed up her situation. "Jody's pregnancy brought up everything from a lot of Sunday mornings and tested all of us. Jody's parents have shown their total love for her and their respect for what she thinks. When they said they would take care of her baby they meant every word of it. Don't think badly about the young man here, either. He's a fine boy. Nor do I think Jody is at fault. She wanted to be like other women."

Families like Jody's are not often seen in the clinic. When parents communicate openly with their daughter, respect her views, and support her mature choices, there is theoretically very little reason for her to suffer an unwanted pregnancy. If, as sometimes happens anyway, women in these families do become pregnant, their family relationships are strong enough to weather the problems that result.

The disappearing window of adolescence need not be a threatening or disruptive experience for either parent or child. Parental understanding of their daughter's early maturity can be both unifying to the family and preventive of many of the problems of becoming a responsible adult, unwanted pregnancy being only one.

It is important for parents to state their values and beliefs honestly and frankly, offering the deepest insights of their own personal experiences. There isn't a need to *agree* with the young woman's values or choices. Daughters can value parental opinions highly, even if they are upset when they hear them, so long as there is never any doubt that their parents gave those opinions honestly, with basic respect and affection. This is the very basis of support into emotionally secure adulthood.

Parental acceptance and realistic communication can

also offer an emerging woman self-acceptance and additional confidence in handling the new experiences she will encounter. Simply put, she can ask questions, request help, share new and powerful feelings, admit doubts, and anticipate an exciting adulthood. This can build strong parent-child relationships that can last through the lifetime of both parents and children.

The key to parental success lies in helping children assume responsibility for their lives as they become ready for it. The adolescent's closing "window of time" admits less light. If a parent's strongest illumination is provided, honest and realistic communication has a powerful and gratifying effect on *both* sides of the window. Families who achieve this have few reasons for their daughters to have an unwanted pregnancy. It happens occasionally, as in Jody's case, but not because of lack of communication or understanding.

It is when parental support and assistance are missing, as in Michelle's family, that unwanted pregnancies occur with seemingly unavoidable regularity. The daughters of these families have the greatest need for the clinic, and an abortion is just the latest of many problems for these young women.

Today, personal desires and choices are too honest to be cranked out of idealistic formulas. Each child is different, just as each parent and family are unique. When people respect and accept each other as the complex, constantly growing adults that they are from the young teenage years onward, family bonds strong enough to last a lifetime become possible.

The Dolly Dilemma. Even the most sincere family support doesn't solve all problems. Some sexually active young women aren't mature enough to understand or listen to their parents when their parents are right. One situation that we see with disturbing frequency is the dilemma of the very young woman who wants to keep her pregnancy.

Donna made a surprising first impression because she was very thin and certainly did not have the physical development that people imagine when they consider a young woman who is pregnant. This twelve-year-old was in my office with her parents because they had been through counseling and reached a dead end. Donna wanted a dolly—a living, breathing, crying, wet-in-its-pants dolly that talks. As I looked at her, Donna was quiet and appeared somewhat nervous at being in a doctor's office, but occasionally betrayed an unmistakable curiosity about what was happening around her.

Her father was also very quiet, though deeply concerned about what was happening. He felt totally out of place and buried himself in a large armchair off to the side.

Donna's mother was neither withdrawn nor domineering. She had an obvious, close relationship with her daughter. The two of them sat together on the couch, and Donna seemed pleased whenever her mother touched her reassuringly. I asked her mother to explain the situation to me as she saw it.

"Donna is an active, healthy twelve-year-old girl. She's not one of those problem kids you read about. She's happy at home and does everything she's supposed to do around the house. Of course, she knows how she got pregnant, but hardly went looking for it, I can tell you. That whole story is pretty involved and I'd rather not go into it, if that's all right. One of our relatives is pretty sick. We've seen to it that he's watched carefully when he's around children and he's getting treated for his problems."

Donna tried to pretend that she wasn't listening. She looked at a painting of a lion cub on the wall over my desk.

"Anyway," her mother said, "Charlie and I nearly

died when we found out that Donna is pregnant. She's too young to become a mother. I'm sure you see that, right? But we have a problem with her. She thinks that actually having her own baby would be just fine." She looked nervously at Donna, who responded with the half-pleased, half-determined look of any twelve-year old who has absolutely decided on the toy she wants for Christmas.

"We explained to her," she went on. "I mean we really did explain *everything* to her. First of all, having a baby isn't that much fun. And then taking care of it. And how it would change her life while she was growing up. But Donna said to us, 'Well, you can help.' "

Donna seemed pleased that the presentation was fair and maintained her aloofness and quiet determination. Her father had been fidgeting nervously, and at this point said, "Are we really in a bad mess? We're ready to sign whatever papers you need, but my brother, who takes care of my legal things, said it might not be that simple. He's a good lawyer but I don't think he knows what he's talking about in this case. He said that it's the same as when a kid can get an abortion on her own if she wants. That's really terrible, but it isn't the same if Donna wants to keep her baby, is it? Wouldn't that be a mess!"

Donna's father leaned forward, looked me right in the eye, and said, "We know what she needs and now are you going to sit there and tell me we can't make her do it?"

I took a deep breath before answering. I had to tell them that there are indeed serious legal problems. Then I said that it would be important in either event for Donna to feel that she understood this decision because she would be thinking about it for years. I have to confess that I was uncomfortable with the sound of my words. I was making the kind of noises that an expert makes, and it sounded silly. But this child was eleven weeks pregnant and I knew that trying to get through to her within the next seven days might prove futile. The almost impossible trick would be to do so without trampling her feelings altogether and damaging her sense of self-esteem for years to come.

With such a short period of time left, I called out the reserves. It didn't take long before my chief counselor was involved in the problem. There was also some help from the family's minister, who was already aware of what was happening. A phone call to him proved very quickly that he was also more concerned about the emotional effects of commanding this child to do one thing or another than the peculiar reverse twist of the law.

I hoped that with the extra time they could put into it my counselors could be of real help, despite the fact that our basic attitude is never to try to talk anyone into or out of a decision regarding abortion. All these people worked together closely for many weeks and I had several conversations with Donna, trying to draw her into a deeper realization of what the next several years might be like for her, one way or the other.

It was no use. Donna wanted her dolly.

When the next month had passed and I had heard nothing more from this family I felt badly because it was clear what was happening. I couldn't suppress the rather bitter thought that only the most emotional antiabortion people could be pleased.

Under the law, not only are parents helpless to prevent a young woman from having an abortion if she wants one, they also cannot make her have an abortion if she doesn't want one. Our experience at the clinic is that most parents are angry at the Supreme Court decision allowing every young woman to have an abortion—until their teenage daughter becomes pregnant. Then they bring their daughter to the clinic immediately, and insist that she have an abortion, which we never perform unless it is the decision of the pregnant young woman herself. If, on the other hand, the young woman wants to keep the pregnancy, parents suddenly discover themselves on the opposite side of the fence—angry at the Supreme Court because they can't force their daughter to have an abortion.

The sexual adulthood of teenage women is a sharp knife that cuts deep, especially if a young woman is not mature enough to make a wise decision when presented with the facts of her situation—or if she keeps her pregnancy to hurt her parents. Donna is not alone. Thousands of young women like her are learning what it means to live with a real-live dolly. It is a lesson that their families can hardly be expected to appreciate.

"One for the Road" in Separation or Divorce

Stacey closed her eyes and let her head fall back until it was motionless, as if it were poised to drop off her shoulders. She took a slow, deep breath then let the air sigh out. When she sat up and looked at me, tears were in her eyes. "Isn't a divorce enough?" she asked. "Now I'm pregnant. I'm so mad I could die!"

This predicament has come to be known as "one for the road" pregnancy. That phrase was invented as a joke by one of my counselors, but with the passage of time it became apparent that it wasn't a joke at all. It is a real phenomenon that occurs often enough and includes enough different kinds of women that we came to accept it as a valid social finding. As we investigated further, we learned that it has a definite cause.

Stacey, like so many other women who are in the middle of a divorce or separation, described a wave of overwhelming emotion that she shared with her soon-to-be ex-husband. It resulted in intercourse. As she put it, "In a way it was beautiful. We made love once more and I broke down and cried in his arms. I was sorry for how much we lost from when we were first married."

We have found that couples who separate without animosity, as well as those who openly hate each other, feel this last wave and frequently respond to it. They don't always respond sexually. They sometimes do so with an unexpected act of generosity, such as reaching an amicable settlement in an evening after weeks of fighting. No matter how they respond, this represents a kind of personal cleaning of the slate, a compensation for whatever contribution they made to the relationship's problems. This wave of emotion helps end the relationship decently, and frees the person's conscience for the first steps of a new life.

When the one for the road encounter is sexual, the woman is extremely vulnerable to pregnancy. This last farewell, or perhaps several intense farewells, can easily occur after a long interval of no physical contact at all. The woman is not apt to have continued birth control pills or have contraceptive paraphernalia handy, except if she has an IUD.

In marriages where the physical relationship is very strong, it can even continue after a divorce. One of the more extreme cases of this took me by surprise one day, when a well-dressed twenty-nine-year-old explained her reasons for wanting an abortion. She had not been able to stop sleeping with her first husband, though they had divorced six years before and both of them had remarried. This woman was understandably unhappy. She wanted a child with her second husband, but she just didn't know whose child she was carrying. I asked her if the abortion would mean she would end the relationship with her first husband. She lowered her eyes and never gave me an answer.

An unwanted pregnancy is always a difficult experience, and one in the middle of a separation or a divorce almost always turns a bad situation into a catastrophe. The worse the troubles between two people, the bigger the crisis caused by the pregnancy. It is easy for someone not involved in the breakup of a relationship to say that an abortion might not be necessary because the marital problems might be worked out. Certainly, a few marriages are begun and others are preserved, at least on paper, because of an existing child or an unexpected pregnancy. In the honesty of sincere discussion with the counselors, however, the most common reaction is, "I've already had enough problems. I don't want to put up with this bad relationship for the rest of my life. Getting pregnant right now was just a stupid mistake."

There is a valuable lesson in this. The need for birth control in a marriage that is over continues until the divorce is final and perhaps even longer than that. At the very least, a supply of condoms, foam, or a diaphragm should be handy, in the event it is needed. The pain of an unwanted pregnancy in the middle of a divorce or separation is so great that it is well worth continuing birth control.

Medical Failures: A Too-frequent Cause

Too many unwanted pregnancies are caused by the mistakes of physicians—a close estimate is just over 10 percent of all the women who have an abortion at my clinic. I've spoken to both individual doctors and groups of physicians about this problem. Their reaction ranges from antagonism, to defensiveness, to sincere concern.

The more antiabortion a doctor is, the more antagonistic his response is likely to be. One physician I have known for years was solidly programed against abortion in childhood, before he even knew what the word meant.

He's a heavyset, back-thumping kind of guy, with rather large hands for an obstetrician. He believed that every pregnancy is a marvelous contribution to God and country, and even discouraged contraception. He went through life never realizing that his attitudes were responsible for a shocking number of women having abortions, the very thing he opposed.

On the other hand, the more sincere the physician the more anxious he is to learn about my disturbing message, and immediately correct any deficiencies in his practice. I'm very happy to say that this includes the great majority of doctors with whom I've spoken. Even a convention of the American College of Obstetricians and Gynecologists came to recognize this problem. Their response to my speech was neither applause nor rejection. It was thoughtful silence. Afterward, I was surrounded by physicians who wanted to discuss it further.

A minority of respectable doctors, however, reacted defensively. "I don't even like abortion," one of these doctors said. "I'm liberal enough to know that this is sometimes necessary, but I wouldn't do anything to contribute to it. Anyway," he continued, looking at me sharply, "you're on pretty shaky ground when you start saying doctors are responsible for anything. In fact, you sound pretty damned irresponsible."

It doesn't give me any joy at all to complain about the mistakes of a few of my fellow physicians. Most doctors try as hard as they can to do the right and proper things for their patients. But these problems must be discussed because my clinic brings to light not hundreds but thousands of women who have found themselves forced—by physicians who had all good intent to the contrary—into the painful decision for abortion.

The need for abortion exists, but anything that can prevent this need should be done. Without question, *all* physicians should assist in prevention, since this is the professional group to which the public turns for help. Doctors have the training and obligation to prevent medical problems, not cause them.

The Four Most Common Mistakes of Doctors. I refused to believe the following problems existed when I first opened the clinic. I started to listen seriously only when patients reported them time after time. Once I opened my ears a variety of complaints about doctors forced me to study the pregnancies that turned out to be routinely caused by some physicians. I must reemphasize that these are the mistakes of a *minority* of doctors. There is no question that most physicians are dedicated to the overall well-being of their patients.

The unwanted pregnancies that result from frank misinformation come first. Confusion about medical facts is bad enough when it is passed back and forth over coffee by women who discuss how they think their bodies work. It is downright harmful when it comes from the authoritative voice of a doctor, who should know better. Every single week pregnant women explain that they haven't been using contraceptives because their doctors told them it would be difficult, if not impossible, for them to become pregnant.

By the time I saw her, at the age of twenty-four, Dina had been to five different doctors, and all of them had told her the same thing: the combination of a retroverted uterus and irregular periods might make it very difficult for her to become pregnant. She had a diaphragm, but only used it occasionally because she believed she wouldn't get pregnant when she didn't want to use it. Eventually, the odds caught up with her.

Dina expressed her feelings with some bitterness. "I don't think doctors know what they're talking about. I put too much faith in what they told me, and now I have to decide what to do about this pregnancy." Dina also said that she was angry with herself for not knowing that she really could become pregnant. She had trusted doctors who, as she put it, "didn't have to deal with the results of their mistake."

When a physician says to a woman, "It is difficult for you to become pregnant," the patient often *hears* the doctor say, "You can't become pregnant." To clear up this misunderstanding a doctor should say, "There is still a chance you can get pregnant, so you need to use birth control." Simply put, the doctor must emphasize the fact that this woman can become pregnant, not how difficult this is for her.

A variety of reasons are given to women why pregnancy is unlikely, among them are having irregular periods, a tipped or retroverted uterus, having fibroids on the uterus, only one ovary or only one tube, the possibility of endometriosis, or the presence of a systemic disease such as diabetes, tuberculosis, and so forth.

It is true that any of these conditions may contribute to infertility. But infertility only means difficulty in becoming pregnant. It does not mean sterility, which is the impossibility of pregnancy.

Infertility and sterility are not interchangeable words. Many patients think they are. This is a fact all physicians should recognize and make clear. Women who have any of these conditions and don't realize that they are still fertile should be advised about contraception immediately.

The golden rule, which must be emphasized by every physician to every woman, is simple: *Every woman with at least one ovary, one tube, and a uterus is capable of becoming pregnant.* Any physician or patient who neglects this is courting an unexpected and perhaps unwanted pregnancy.

The second serious mistake arises when a doctor removes a woman from one kind of contraceptive without recommending that she start another form of contraception *immediately*. Several times a week I hear a story like Annie's. She called her doctor with a minor complaint, that she had a few extra pounds of weight which she suspected might come from retaining fluids while on the pill. She was told, "Well, just stop using it."

When I met Annie seven weeks later we had a chance to discuss that conversation. "Did your doctor suggest that you use something else?" I asked.

"No. He just said stop the pill."

"Did you ask for help in establishing another kind of birth control?" I continued, still wondering why she was pregnant.

"Yes, but he said, 'Let's just watch and see. Check with me in three months.'"

"What did he say when you turned up pregnant?"

"He said, 'That's terrible. You knew you should be careful.'"

Ridiculous as this conversation sounds, it happens too often to be funny. A related mistake that is also common occurs when a physician feels a patient should have a "rest" from the pill. My counselors have probed to find out why the pregnant women they see were taken off the pill. To the best of our knowledge, in most cases it was an arbitrary decision by a doctor. There wasn't any specific problem, complication, or even nausea. Perhaps the real reason is that this "rest" relieves the doctor's conscience because of the scare stories about the pill.

If this is a questionable problem for a doctor's conscience, a larger, more certain problem can occur if he doesn't recommend an alternative form of contraception. Many women whose bodies became pregnant instead of "resting" have told the counselors that they understood that their system takes time to get back to normal, so they should have been safe soon after going off the pill. This is an obvious myth because a woman can miss one or two pills and become pregnant right away. It is the same as soon as she abandons *any* form of birth control.

Every physician who removes a patient from one method of birth control has a responsibility to stress the use of another form of contraception immediately. There is a real possibility that if he does not, his patient might wind up at an abortion clinic. Nor does the case have to end there. Some of these pregnant women have said that they wish they could sue their doctors for prescribing a "rest" from the pill. A couple of women have even suggested suing for trauma, resulting from a trying abortion related to the omission of alternative contraceptive counseling.

The third common problem is the lack of time spent by physicians with their patients when they prescribe contraceptives. This causes insufficient understanding, and the patient does not use her birth control method effectively. I feel somewhat embarrassed by the necessity of reminding some of my peers that giving medication has little value without the proper instructions and follow-up that must accompany it.

Why does this happen? The main reason is the mistaken assumption by physicians that patients already know the significant facts about the various forms of birth control. Most doctors have discussed and recommended contraceptives to thousands of women over many years. It is easy for them to forget that each new woman has a real need to be treated like the very first woman requiring medical help in this area.

A doctor's office time is short. It is easy to skip a five-minute discussion on which form of birth control is best for that particular woman, and how she must use it if it is to be effective. It's true that three other patients are waiting to be seen and prescribing birth control doesn't appear as urgent as a patient with vaginal bleeding in the next room. But the impact of an unwanted pregnancy outweighs this viewpoint. *The prescription of birth control is not an insignificant moment for either the physician or the patient.*

Many of the clinic's patients have possessed a diaphragm but only had the vaguest idea of what to do with it. At that level of knowledge, a diaphragm's only value is as a bedroom frisbee. Even among women who can insert a diaphragm properly, how many have been advised that this should be used with contraceptive jelly and should be left in place for eight hours after intercourse?

The use of the pill demands that the patient be instructed as thoroughly as possible. The potential side effects of the pill have to be explained. Quite a large number of women have abandoned birth control pills in panic upon reading a critical newspaper story or when slight spotting or light bleeding has occurred, only to turn up at the clinic a short time later.

The crowning problem, on the patient's part, is not insisting upon complete contraceptive instructions. She should not be afraid. These few moments have an overwhelming impact on her life. The anxiety she will encounter with an unwanted pregnancy will be much greater than any discomfort she may feel interrupting a busy doctor to have her birth control properly prescribed.

The fourth common mistake of physicians does not cause a pregnancy. It delays confirming a pregnancy and this may compound the problems of a woman who must have an abortion. There is nothing nice, understanding, or forgiving I can say about the physician who responds to a woman's question of whether she is pregnant with only a question on the phone about her last menstrual period, or having his nurse run a pregnancy test. A pelvic examination must be done as soon as possible. When an unwanted pregnancy isn't confirmed until the second trimester, a woman's expense and emotional turmoil are aggravated substantially, as we have observed.

"That's impossible," I'm often told. "I just had a negative pregnancy test in my doctor's office two weeks ago."*

Marcia's case illustrates that this laxity exists even with women who reach for closer supervision by their physician. Marcia lost all her composure and started crying when I informed her that she was fourteen weeks pregnant. "I can't be this far along," she said. "I had a period two months ago and marked it on my calendar. But I called my doctor. I really did, because my breasts were getting swollen and I was sick in the mornings, and he knew another pregnancy might kill me . . . he was the one who told me that. But he said there's no point in checking until I miss two periods. I don't understand how I can be this much pregnant with the bleeding."

The fact of the matter is that not all bleeding is menstrual bleeding, though it may appear to be so. Bleeding that looks like a period may occur early in pregnancy. There wasn't any doubt that Marcia was fourteen weeks pregnant. She sat there with the drape across her waist and stared helplessly at the floor. "What am I going to do now? There is just no way I can keep this pregnancy."

Marcia felt upset and betrayed because she had called

---

* Pregnancy tests are not always accurate. False positives and false negatives occur, regardless of the kind of test used. Physicians must stress to their lab assistants that *a pregnancy test performed on a urine specimen without a specific gravity of 1.015 or greater cannot be accepted if the results are negative.* Otherwise, the hormones in the urine which turn a pregnancy test positive may be too diluted to make the test work. In a matter of such great importance, the extra check of the specific gravity of the urine sample must be done *routinely.*

the one physician she really trusted in these matters, and now that her pregnancy was confirmed it was too late to get the help she needed at a clinic. Most of her trauma could have been avoided if her doctor had taken more interest at the moment she first called.

The ease of suction curettage in the first twelve weeks of pregnancy, compared with a more complex and expensive hospital procedure in the second trimester, makes the immediate confirmation of pregnancy medically significant. Even though a physician may have treated a particular woman for years, he probably does not know her current views on having another child. Doctors can no longer assume that every potential pregnancy is a blessing until they have some sign of this from the woman herself. Physician responsibility for confirming a pregnancy must be taken seriously, so that women who do not cherish the onset of a pregnancy can minimize the extent of the tragedy they face.

Nonphysician Physicians. It is shocking to hear again and again from pregnant women of all ages that they sought professional help in preventing pregnancy and received insults or a lecture on morality instead. Such doctors' offices are a far cry from the place of sanctuary that they should be, where a woman in need can request treatment according to her own emotional, moral, religious, or social needs.

The extensive personal difficulties such an experience can cause are exemplified by Darlene. She was fifteen and in her first year of high school. Nobody would question that she had to be one of the brightest girls in her class. She had the kind of smile that makes toothpaste ads work, and she was very popular. For two years she had been going steady with her boyfriend. He was starting high school, too, and they were considering starting intercourse. They put it off until she could arrange birth control.

All Darlene wanted was the pill. It seemed a lot to go through, making an appointment with a doctor across town, reading a magazine in a strange waiting room for an hour when she was supposed to be in school, then sitting under a towel on a cold table for twenty minutes more. But when the doctor blew in he was breezy and reassuring. He had sandy hair and looked young enough to still know what it was like to have feelings for someone. The pelvic exam and Pap smear weren't that bad, and sitting in his office with her clothes on again was like reaching the other side of a turbulent river.

After some talk about allergies and whether she still had her tonsils, he asked, "Any particular problems?"

"Well, not really," she said. "But I don't want to get pregnant."

"You don't want to get pregnant? What do you mean?"

For a moment Darlene thought he was kidding, but his friendly grin was gone and he suddenly seemed more like a grumpy school principal. "I just don't want to get pregnant," she said, and was a hair away from making a dash for the door.

"Listen," he said, "you shouldn't be fooling around . . . it's a long time before you'll be married. When I was dating I want to tell you I'd never marry any girl I slept with. You don't want to wind up single, maybe with a child to take care of, and probably with venereal disease, too."

Darlene was halfway between crying and getting mad. "It's not like that," she said.

"Don't tell me what it's like," the kindly doctor replied. "I've been through this with hundreds of you kids. If it's the pill you want, forget it. I'm not going to do anything to help turn you into a tramp. You look too nice. And this little talk will be the best thing that ever happened to you."

It was almost a week before Darlene could tell her boyfriend about this experience, because she was that upset about it. They tried prophylactics twice then switched to foam. A girlfriend told her that the foam was supposed to be used after intercourse. Sure enough, she realized that she was pregnant shortly thereafter. All the problems this caused Darlene would take another book to tell.

This young woman decided she wasn't ready to become a mother. The idea of abortion upset her, but she had her pregnancy terminated. The remarks and veiled insults of some family members and supposed friends didn't help her much either. She was offered birth control pills at the time of her abortion. At first she didn't want to accept them because she didn't want anyone at the clinic to feel that she was a tramp, like that doctor did. Then she thought of the chance of going through another pregnancy and decided to take the prescription.

Darlene's life settled down and she got back to normal over the next six months, until she had to refill her prescription for pills. She just couldn't face that mess again, and about a year later her tragedy repeated itself—she became pregnant again.

Few of the doctors on a moral crusade come on as strong as the one who "treated" Darlene, but these physicians cause considerable numbers of women to suffer the pains of an unwanted pregnancy, even when their intentions are good. At the clinic we see their failures, not their successes, and their failure rate is higher than for any of the other kinds of physician-caused pregnancies.

Certainly, no doctor should be required to separate his philosophy or judgment from the counsel he offers. But in cases where he cannot in good conscience offer a patient medical assistance in line with the *patient's* needs, he *should* refer her to a physician who will help her. In my view, medicine is a helping profession, not a seat from which one can direct the morals of patients in need. No physician has the *medical* right to refuse both help and referral, because that refusal may cause his patient an unwanted pregnancy.

There is a difference between many doctors' public statements and their private practices. In the privacy of consultation rooms the majority of physicians offer compassion, interest, and professionalism worthy of the highest standards of medicine. Overtly, this majority is nearly completely silent. As in most controversies, the noisy minority attracts the most attention.

Increasing numbers of physicians have adopted the attitude that they themselves have no interest in providing abortion services, but they will respect and indirectly assist their patients in securing an abortion when it is needed. Even if this is restricted to the silence of private practices, it is a major shift for conservative physicians. It indicates that the helping values of medicine have strength and vitality, that the real needs of women are understood by the majority of doctors.

Government Contributions to Unwanted Pregnancies

What does the government have to do with unwanted pregnancies that result in abortions? What does it have to do with large numbers of personal and community tragedies that occur in this area? Most people think that the government affects people's lives through laws that are passed and judgments that are rendered. In reality, laws, decisions, and bureaucratic policies are only a part of the way government can affect people.

Consider Eleanor, who was twenty-six and facing her

seventh pregnancy. This young redhead was attractive, bright, and unquestionably fertile. Theoretically, she could work in any number of jobs not requiring too much specialized training. Because she needed the income, she had held a great number of jobs, but they lasted for short periods of time. It always seemed that pregnancy or a problem related to childbearing would catch up with her. Once all that nausea or ill health began, there went another job.

She had two children and one miscarriage in an early marriage; then her husband disappeared. She had another child while living with a man for several years. He had odd jobs and helped support the first two. They had always wanted to get married some day, but realistically they could do better collecting unemployment compensation and welfare. Neither he nor Eleanor enjoyed the idea of taking advantage of the government. It was just a question of getting by. One day, he left as well.

Eleanor was treated well at the health department and the family services offices. Over the years she had become well known and liked by the staffs. They helped her try just about every form of birth control available, but each one brought its own problems and sooner or later she turned up pregnant again. The first crisis came when the family planning division of the health department had to cut back the time and services it could offer because of the lack of funding. This young woman needed specialized care and personal attention by a gynecologist if she were to prevent pregnancy, but that care was becoming progressively more difficult to get.

Her next crisis arose when she had to be admitted to the emergency room of the local hospital for a severe infection in her tubes caused by gonorrhea. These expenses were covered by Medicaid but even they might have been prevented. The little penny culture medium bottles employed in screening for gonorrhea were no longer used by the health department. They were discontinued to cut costs.

Medicaid paid for terminationg her next two pregnancies but those led to a crisis, also. A public health medical assistant decided to do society a favor by giving Eleanor an impressive lecture about all the citizens and people in government who were tired of paying for her abortions, and that if she ever got pregnant again they would probably cut off all of her government assistance. Eleanor went into a panic. She tried to abort herself and wound up in the hospital again with a severe pelvic infection.

The crowning absurdity was that during her last three pregnancies Eleanor had tried to arrange for a tubal ligation. She decided that physically, emotionally, and economically she was in no condition to ever want another pregnancy. She didn't care whether or not the government would pay for the delivery or assist with the financial support of additional children for eighteen years. She evaluated her needs herself and felt that she had all the pregnancies and children she wanted.

Her attempts to pursue sterilization failed. She was told that she was much too young and all women under forty should preserve their ability to become pregnant. Anyway, funds were limited, some physicians might sympathize with her but didn't accept Medicaid cases, and the paperwork hassle of arranging for sterilization was so great it wasn't worth the battle. Unfortunately, all these things, other than the age nonsense, were true to a very great extent.

Not all of Eleanor's problems could have been prevented with more realistic government priorities and interest. But many of them could have been made less severe and others could have been avoided altogether. With the exception of the occasional oddball likely to pop up in any organization, governmental or otherwise, most of the people who tried to help Eleanor cared very much for her welfare. They were hampered severely by cutbacks in areas that were critical to her safety as well as that of hundreds of thousands of women across the country. Thousands of social services reach for help from the federal dollar with varying degrees of justification. I must make the plea for improved priorities and expanded help in this area on the basis of its major impact in the lives of many women who are otherwise trapped into becoming baby machines against their wills, or choosing repeated abortions.

Current bureaucratic policies feed on themselves and forget the patient. Millions of dollars are spent each year for the purely paper function of comprehensive health planning councils, for example. These are also known as health systems agencies. They employ social workers, health planners, administrators, secretaries, and others who direct the time and energies of responsible people in every community of this country, talking about the delivery of health care. These groups review the expansion of medical programs and approve or disapprove eligibility for financial support of the services and facilities that hospitals and physicians in a community feel are necessary. They play a massive bureaucratic game in the name of saving money by avoiding duplicated services, at least on a theoretical basis. Of the millions of dollars spent on these exercises, little benefits the forgotten person, the patient.

The Public Health Dilemma. Local health departments have come of age in doing the best they can to offer contraceptive counseling and help women avoid pregnancies they don't want. But in the midst of attempting to prevent problems, these agencies suffer from generations-old inhibitions about facing the need for contraception squarely and funding it adequately. The same kinds of people with the same kinds of private philosophies still fight prevention of problem pregnancies just as they do the provision of safe and adequate abortion. Their influence is constantly felt throughout government health care agencies.

The government establishes its priorities of help to the people by being responsive to the needs of the people. So far so good. Problems arise when responsiveness to the many becomes a matter of influence by a few. The unfairness of interest and funding comes about so frequently because those with the greatest needs are usually those with the least influence.

Political influence is not just a question of making wealthy campaign contributions. It is a question of having the time, energy, and know-how, over and above the demands of daily survival, to press personal opinions and philosophies on the government in the form of letters, telegrams, and meetings for one cause or another. Eleanor, like so many women, needs personal assistance in preventing problems and coping with the crises of her life. The idea of writing a letter to her congressman or hunting up a meeting to explain her needs would impress her as an exercise in futility. And so, her voice is rarely, if ever, heard.

The picture of an overfed matron or a suit-and-tie man parading up and down in front of the state capitol with placards saying "Abortion Is Immoral" would strike Eleanor as silly, unfeeling, and unfair. But these people, their placards, letters, and meetings, do have a profound effect on the legislators who write the laws. They tend to respond to the loudest knocks on their doors.

I've found it a very interesting exercise to ask public health administrators and politicians why there should be such a hassle over a woman's getting a tubal ligation if she feels that she never wants to have another pregnancy. The answer is almost universally the same.

"Well, you can't let people have everything they want just because they want it."

"Do you think that women make the decision not to have any more children lightly?"

"No, not usually."

"Do you think that women who don't want more children should continue to be exposed to pregnancy and then have to decide on and probably go through an abortion if they become pregnant?"

"No."

"Do you think that there is a greater public expense in helping a woman to be sterilized or in allowing her to be faced with additional unwanted pregnancies and paying for abortions, deliveries, and all the support required thereafter?"

"Obviously, it would cost less to sterilize women who want it."

"Then why is there all this hassle?"

"Because you can't do what people want just because they want it."

This conversation exposes a basic attitude that needs to be rectified. The attitude still persists that the primary value of a woman is to have babies and that it is the sacred obligation of society in general and the government in particular to do anything in its power to maintain that state of affairs. Most responsible men and women would label that attitude "total nonsense." Yet this total nonsense does persist and does exert its influence in the responses as well as the legislation affecting the everyday lives of people.

This attitude makes it very difficult for many public health workers even to discuss the immediate problems of an unwanted pregnancy with their patients openly and honestly. The fear of going against the personal objections to abortion referral of someone higher in the line of government bureaucracy has translated itself into a very palpable fear of losing one's job.

The Medicaid Controversy. Women with severe financial problems have been able to find access to abortion through the government assistance of Medicaid. During this time the opponents of abortion have launched a massive effort to influence legislators at the national and state level. One of their main goals is to stop any federal expenditures to these services. A direct attack on Medicaid was based on the idea that since some people don't like the idea of abortion, federal funds should not be available to people who need it.

This tactic succeeded, for instance, in the 1976 Health, Education, and Welfare funding bill. The money was desperately needed and there was a great deal of pressure to get the bill out of committee and on the books. The Hyde Amendment was added to this bill as a rider. It said that the government would not pay any funds for abortion other than cases where the life or health of the mother was at stake. Many congressmen and senators resented this rider, but the pressure to get the whole bill passed was greater than the need to clean the trash off it.

In June 1977 the Supreme Court ruled that states do not have the obligation to use Medicaid funds for the indigent requiring abortion. This decision was received as a massive setback to honoring individual rights and the personal judgments of poor people. It was labeled discriminatory by many, but that label was no help. Although the letter of constitutionality may have been correct, the net effects could be only harmful.

The real problems of an unwanted pregnancy for someone who can barely support an existing family have never interested the opponents of abortion. Poverty-stricken families live with hunger, few job openings for

192 A WOMAN'S CHOICE

the unskilled, too little pay for those who can find work, and a lack of society's interest in this fate. Ending the medical support for dealing with unwanted pregnancy must result in more neglect of the emotional, social, and financial needs of the poor. It is a virtual guarantee that their families will be large, their struggle for day-to-day survival severe, and their condemnation to another generation of poverty a good possibility.

If compulsory pregnancy for the poor becomes reality, an unwanted pregnancy gives a poor woman only one of two choices. In about half the cases her choice will be to keep the pregnancy and raise the child at further government expense—in the first year alone it is ten to fifteen times the cost of an abortion. The only reason the cost to government is mentioned is that one of the phony arguments brought up repeatedly is that the government should save money by not spending public dollars to terminate pregnancies. This argument is blatantly ridiculous.

The other alternative to poor women without government support is the continuation of the horrible examples of the past: self-induced abortion or women who subject themselves to butchery by untrained people.

Nationwide Fears. I must nail a charge of careless judgment and perhaps irresponsibility at the door of the Food and Drug Administration. This is a massive agency with direct influence on the practice of medicine and even greater influence on the thinking and fears of millions of people. Hundreds of women seen in my clinic alone have discarded their pills in a moment of fear unrelated to any specific medical problem, because warnings are released for publication without adequate, reasonable, or truthful perspective.

The damage caused by the FDA is not limited to birth control pills, nor is its mischief limited to warnings.

Many valuable medications are taken from physicians'
hands and denied to the public for barely justifiable reasons. The most widely known case was the outrageous ban
on saccharin. Despite generations of beneficial use, saccharin was challenged by the FDA because they felt that a
person who drinks eight hundred cans of diet soda every
day of his life *might* develop cancer. No mention was made
of the harmful effects of an equivalent amount of real
sugar, or the injury to the many diabetics and dieters who
depend on the sugar substitute. Similarly, the FDA banned
half the forms of birth control pills. In light of this record,
there is no reason to suppose that one morning the FDA
may not make an announcement and summarily wipe out
the rest.

Pick up any of hundreds of articles about the pill ultimately referable to positions taken by the Food and
Drug Administration. How many of these articles imply
that women taking birth control pills face the real danger
of imminent death? Most of them. How many of these
articles make clear that the risk of pregnancy or abortion
is greater than the risk of using the pill? Virtually none.
How many labels in these contraceptives inform the public of the full picture of contraceptive safety plus the
risk of terminating or continuing an unexpected pregnancy caused by a less reliable method of birth control?
Virtually none. How many FDA officials are willing to
admit publicly that the impact of the publicity about the
pill has hurt the public more than helped it? Virtually
none. The next question must follow. Does the public
have good reason to wonder if the trust it puts in the FDA
is misplaced?

Alerting the public to potential dangers of the pill or
anything else is of itself no problem. Properly done it is
commendable. Without total perspective, however, more
harm is done than good. I must make the plea that the

FDA be constrained to follow nothing but complete and full disclosure in every pronouncement to the public and to the medical profession as well. And this restraint should extend far beyond matters dealing with contraceptives alone.

How Can the Government Help? Other than making and enforcing laws, the greatest power government has is in disseminating information. The government has the ear of the people constantly. It has the attention of institutions such as schools, hospitals, health departments, public and private social agencies, and the interest of all professional groups including physicians, nurses, social workers, and counselors. The manner in which any topic is discussed and the recommendations suggested have an immediate and overwhelming impact. Quite often, the federal government does not have to force attention or even compliance. Because the first exists, the second has instant momentum.

A letter from the FDA may be opened with suspicion by physicians, but it will be opened and read. If that letter were to contain factual information about oral contraceptives based on a perspective that included the large numbers of women for whom it is safe, and the letter were to indicate that this perspective was available to the public as well, then many physicians would not have to maintain a position of needless overdefensiveness in prescribing this contraceptive. Many physicians who advise patients to "take a rest from the pill" do so only out of defensiveness and with the fear of being attacked for not being cautious enough. I can cite literally hundreds of examples where physicians summarily discontinued the pill from use by a patient because of the slightest hint of any problem at all, whether related to the pill or not. The numbers of unwanted pregnancies that result from these actions are much greater than anyone imagines. Government communication can teach as well as intimidate. It can give assurance as well as create doubt. It can and should solidify mutual trust between a patient and her physician, and provide a reliably authoritative framework within which patient needs can be met on the basis of truth instead of fear.

Literature, brochures, and information dealing with preventing unwanted pregnancies would be opened, studied, and possibly used if they came from the Department of Health, Education, and Welfare. School counselors, parents groups, ministers, and others are very eager for factual guidance and help in dealing with the sexual problems of the young. That concern must be channeled into rational understanding to avoid many sexual problems of teenagers.

I'm not recommending that the government should make a frontal assault and carry the banner of sex education in the schools. This is a topic that has been clouded with misunderstanding for a long time. In the way of a personal experiment, ask parents what "sex education in the schools" means to them. You may be shocked to learn that parents fear that sex education implies no more than teaching youngsters how to enjoy sex. On the other hand, ask high school students what sex education in the schools might or should mean. You may well learn that their average response refers to ways to avoid problems, either physical or emotional.

Teenagers make comments like, "Everybody talks about not getting venereal disease, but I don't know what to do because the only thing I've been told is, 'Be careful,' or, 'See your doctor if you have any problems.'" They say they get the same treatment when it comes to avoiding pregnancy. Alicia, who was pregnant, said, "All I was told was not to get pregnant until I'm ready for it. Lots of luck.

That wasn't any help at all."

Valid information on all these subjects would be respected and welcomed by PTA groups, churches, fraternal and civic organizations, and other people who assist teenagers in growing up, all of whom are constantly looking for meaningful subjects of discussion and new ways to help. There is so much that could be done and so much that is not being done that the government must share responsibility for a significant amount of today's unwanted pregnancies because of the sin of omission.

The needs for abortion can never be legislated away. History has proven that. But those needs can be lessened by preventing problem pregnancies and these are only a few of the specific steps that can be taken in that direction.

I do feel that a very constructive step would be the establishment at the federal level of an advisory commission on reproductive medicine. This commission might have reporting responsibility to the head of HEW. It should coordinate and disseminate the best material on prevention and care among all the professionals, institutions, and providers of medical and social care. Its ultimate objective would be to decrease the need for abortion by expanding the measures that prevent this problem from occurring.

As it is today, there are countless major and minor study groups, councils, organizations and the like dedicated to gathering information on these subjects, competing for federal dollars, and yielding an inefficient mess of academic good intentions and overlapping functions. Even very valuable findings rarely reach professionals actually dealing with patients. The distribution of correlated information is a most important area in which such a commission may take the lead.

The commission could also help establish priorities for expenditure of funds and more constructive policies dealing with contraception and sterilization. It should direct its energies to increasing the public's access to advisory and assistance services in all of these areas. It should not be drowned in the protocol of paralyzing philosophical argument or sabotaged by red tape and its findings should be made available directly to the public at large as well as both the executive and legislative branches of government.

These suggestions may seem to be biased because of my particular interest in this area of medicine. But I make the plea that of all areas of medicine, none has a greater impact on such vast numbers of families or touches so many lives. Reproductive medicine has the furthest reaching effects on the quality of life and the economics of life on community, state, and national levels. An unwanted pregnancy is not an isolated problem. This bell tolls long and loudly, extending through a spectrum of personal tragedies, including family instability, personal economic problems, child abuse, aid to dependent children, welfare, personal neglect, alienation, the high level of stress in our society, and crime of all sorts. The phrase "Every pregnancy should be a wanted pregnancy" is much more than a pleasant thought. It is a concept which potentially touches hundreds of lives at a time. It is worthy of recognition and an honest effort at the governmental level. It should be understood and treated for what it is, one of the determiners of the quality of life itself.

10
A NEW DIMENSION OF UNDERSTANDING

"Cry for Help" Pregnancies

A new and dramatic observation at the clinic is that the psychological mechanism that causes attempted suicides is also the basis for several kinds of requests for abortion. An attempted suicide has been recognized for many years as a desperate cry for help. In the clinic we have found that several more kinds of cry for help exist.

Why did Margo try to commit suicide? She was found just in time by her boyfriend in a scene that could have been copied from any of a hundred TV shows. Her apartment was clean and everything in it had been neatly arranged. All her makeup was on. In the middle of this cared-for home she was sprawled, unconscious, on the pillows of her white couch, wearing a fluffy pink nightgown. Her beauty was a shocking contrast to the bright red blood that dribbled down her arms and stained the couch on which she lay.

Margo's boyfriend called the hospital and they rushed her to the emergency room in an ambulance. Margo's parents and minister arrived soon, and found her boyfriend pacing the waiting room.

After a few minutes of treatment, a doctor came out to reassure everyone that with a few bandages, a tetanus shot, and a night's rest she could go home. He waited for the appropriate sighs of relief. Then he gave very careful and detailed instructions how each of the people there could help Margo deal with the undoubtedly great emotional stresses that could lead her to try to take her life.

The doctor did not know Margo's specific problems, but he did know that attempted suicide meant one important thing. It was an overwhelming, desperate cry that revealed the quietest kind of hysteria. She reacted this way because she felt that no one she could confide in really cared enough to help her become happy again. After words and hints and all the obvious signs had failed her, suicide was a last, desperate cry for help.

Few people really want to hurt themselves, but many people find that they are in an intolerable situation from time to time. They may come to feel that they are alone with one or many problems that they don't know how to handle. If they give clues or say they are upset but nobody seems to care, they may consider drastic action. Their initial problems, whatever they may be, become compounded by these feelings of desperation. Then they might consciously or unconsciously take drastic actions.

Susan sat rigidly upright on the edge of the examining table in the clinic. Her legs were tightly crossed and her hands were folded firmly on the towel that covered her lap. Even her lips were set as if to protect her from revealing more than she had to. Her dress, which was rolled up to her waist, matched her large steel blue eyes. The softest thing about her was her hair, which fell to her shoulders in flowing curls. This contrast was the only clue that her excessive control covered emotions that had reached the boiling point inside.

Susan hardly spoke, but her medical records said a great deal. She was sixteen, the daughter of a financially prominent, social register mother and father. The best of everything was constantly offered her and expected from her. Too-frequent treatments at my clinic, starting with an abortion at the age of fourteen and a half, was not one of the advantages her parents enjoyed giving her. She had visited the clinic three times since then for suspected pregnancies, but they proved negative. On this, her fifth visit, her pregnancy test and pelvic exam indicated that she was pregnant for the second time.

"Susan," I said, "this has gone beyond what makes any sense at all. If I'm going to help you, it's time for some straight talk." I held up her file where she couldn't help but look at it. "You're using this place as the center of a psychodrama. If it's too much for you to explain why, you're going to have to go someplace else."

Talking down to this tightly controlled young woman wasn't a safe bet, but the gamble worked. In my office I asked her again, "Why, Susie? Your parents are in the waiting room and they really look like they care for you—"

"They do not!" she interrupted. "And that's the truth. They care about how I look and who I see. Mother's off being a big wheel with her charities and Daddy's forever doing something with his businesses. Even Jonathan, my boyfriend, worries more about how I look than what I really think. He's even like that in bed. He's more concerned about . . . my doing this and that for him than what I feel while we're together.

"You want to know why I come here all the time? Because I don't take my birth control pills—ever. When I come here, my parents jump. All of a sudden, they care about me. It's the only time they do. That's just fine. If I've got to have problems before they're interested in me, I'll show them how many problems I can have!" Susan's face tightened, she dropped her head in her hands, and sobs shook her body.

I called a counselor to take care of Susan while I went out to talk to her parents. They said that she was such a sweet and darling child, but they wondered why she kept winding up at the clinic. In answer to my questions, they admitted, "We should spend more time together, like our family picnic last August, but there is just too much to do, and Lord knows, there's just no young child with more advantages in life."

Susan was surrounded by people, but alone. She had lots of "toys," but little emotional security. In her hands, sex was a powerful weapon that could get her some of the attention she needed. Instead of using the birth control pills her parents had given her, she disregarded them in a desperate attempt to secure their love in the only way she could capture it.

On a conscious level, everyone knows that self-destructiveness does not solve personal problems. But under stress, it is difficult to be rational. Many people have an automatic, unconscious reaction when they are in desperate need: "When I am hurt someone *must* care. If I hurt badly enough, they will care more. I hurt so much already, it doesn't matter how much more it takes to show them."

This reaction is common from childhood through old age. Think of the angry child who refuses to eat dinner even though he is very hungry. Picture a grandmother who doesn't accept a long-wanted invitation to visit her children and grandchildren because she hasn't been invited for too long. Imagine a wife who becomes upset, tearfully yanks out the biggest suitcase, and starts flinging clothes into it, in full view of her children and husband. All of these people really want someone to say, "We love you."

School counselors report a widespread problem with teenage women who repeatedly run away from home even after really concerned parents become overly sensitized to their needs. Patty was a fifteen-year-old who abused her parents' concern so much that her problems and her threats actually dominated the family. She let her parents know that she was often exposed to the possibility of pregnancy, and enjoyed the anxiety and feelings of helplessness she caused them. It delighted her that no one could stop her from getting pregnant, but her abortion was not as satisfying as she had hoped.

Her unquenchable needs had created a destructive force that her parents could no longer accept. After everything they could think of had failed many times, they finally threw up their hands to preserve their sanity. They detached themselves emotionally from Patty. Even though they still meant well and did help her when she needed an abortion, they felt her problems were beyond saving.

Most cry-for-help pregnancies contain elements of self-destructiveness, but they take several distinct forms. The first kind includes women like Susan or Patty who use their sexuality as a weapon against their parents or husbands.

The second kind of cry-for-help pregnancy is so common everyone should recognize it. The red flag of danger, signaling that a woman is playing with self-injury in a desperate attempt to gain compassion, caring, or even interest, is seen in people of all ages. Adults need to be cared about and cared for, just as young women like Susan do. Growing up doesn't eliminate problems, it simply changes them. All people find their problems are easier to face when they receive warmth and support from the people they love.

Olivia was a stable woman in her mid-thirties. Everything in her life was proper and well ordered, from the neatness of her children's clothes to her punctuality at church. Her husband was a steady, dependable sort of man. He spent three nights a week at home, two nights late at the office, and two nights bowling or at the lodge. All of this security was a comfortable cage that was driving Olivia to a quietly frantic state. She felt like a part in a big machine. She needed to feel like a real woman who was important, desired, and more interesting than a refrigerator door. Becoming sloppy, a little late, and careless with this and that were early signs of trouble.

Her husband's reaction didn't help. He began showing flashes of temper when these rough spots first appeared in his home life, which had been smooth enough to require practically no attention. When Olivia began first a few, then many, drinks a day, he'd had it, and summarily shipped her off to a psychiatrist before she lost her grip altogether. He never found time to go with her, but he figured it was her problem, not his.

At the worst possible time in her life, Olivia became careless in one more area. She neglected one, then two, then a whole pack of birth control pills at a time. When I confirmed her pregnancy in my office, her feelings were at the edge of the plank. "I don't know what's going to happen," she said. "I haven't seen Chuck furious that often, but I know he will be now. It was so stupid of me, but everything I do is stupid to him. He may just leave. He's threatened it already. If he does, I don't know . . . I may have an abortion, though I really wouldn't want to. I'd like him to stay. Maybe everything will be all right again."

She looked up with helpless tears, hoping for even a word of assurance. "Do you think they will be?" she asked.

When the counselors ask women why they are pregnant a surprising number of them describe all kinds of problems in their lives. Pregnancy puts these women in a situation where, in effect, they have the chance to say, "I have a big problem, an unwanted pregnancy, and it can't wait ... now that I'm telling you about my problems, look at these others—"

The third kind of cry-for-help pregnancy is an inner scream against fate or life itself. Evelyn was a level-headed woman in her early forties who had raised a son and two daughters to young adulthood. She enjoyed a full life, night classes, tennis, and lots of great sex with her husband. Seven months before she came to the clinic she had a routine examination that revealed a lump in her right breast. Her doctor tried not to alarm her but insisted it be biopsied right away. In that minute, Evelyn felt the ground fall out from under her. She knew that she had cancer, and her life would never be the same.

The surgeon said her operation was a success, but Evelyn couldn't hear his words. Her breast was gone. She was in a daze, and several women who had mastectomies visited her. They helped her more than any doctor, by demonstrating that her life was far from over.

Evelyn wanted to make a comeback from the stiffness in her chest and arm, and the waves of nausea that went along with the radiation treatments. But sex became her biggest problem. After years of luxury on the pill, it was ruled out for medical reasons. She tried an IUD, and unfortunately turned out to be the one woman in ten who has more bleeding and cramps than it was worth. Then the mess of foams, diaphragms, and prophylactics was a galling reminder that nothing was the same.

Her doctor suggested having her tubes tied, but she didn't want to go near an operating room again. For some reason, it upset her when her husband suggested having a vasectomy. Although he felt foolish later, he didn't press the point.

Evelyn had to do something, because she was determined to make a major effort to convince herself that she was still attractive to her husband. They settled on a diaphragm and used it conscientiously. Neither of them could forget her doctor's strict lecture about what a pregnancy could do to increase her breast cancer problems.

They took a weekend vacation to forget everything and help reestablish their relationship. One crazy night that weekend it all became just too much. It was the first time Evelyn felt great since her nightmare began. All she wanted was to be a whole woman again. That night she wanted her stupid diaphragm about as much as she wanted another mastectomy.

Sometime that night fate dealt Evelyn another bad hand; she couldn't stop herself from escaping for a few hours. When I saw her five weeks later, she had an unprintable list of descriptions for herself. She was back in reality, but it was too late.

Evelyn didn't react in anger against a particular person, or out of desperation because of her problems. Hers was a cry of release against the constant suppression of being forced to restrict her life. She acted like a diabetic who, impulsively, has to wolf down a pound of chocolate cake, or a man with an ulcer who suddenly couldn't care if his stomach bleeds, so long as he has one more totally wonderful pepperoni pizza. And what about smokers who can't quit because they have to have one more cigarette?

Cry-for-help pregnancies contain a real danger. A woman's problems can take an unhealthy turn for the worse if her desperate solution is basesd on resentment and frank hostility. If she becomes emotionally detached and doesn't feel the pain of the damage she inflicts on her life, she may bruise herself seriously and batter her family.

This is particularly true for a large percentage of *recurring* unwanted pregnancies, where a woman has gone to the extreme of repeatedly being self-destructive. The outward appearance of all these cries for help may be different, but their basic motivations are the same.

Social Rape: A Nationwide Epidemic?

When most people think of rape they mentally imagine a woman walking down a dark street and being attacked by a sex-starved hoodlum who beats her up, throws her to the ground, tears off her clothes, and forces her to submit to intercourse. The more she struggles and screams, the more he likes what is happening. This criminal has dominated and controlled a woman and received intense sexual gratification at the same time. This is a powerful experience for a man who doesn't have what it takes to establish a relationship with a woman he desires.

This popular image exists because a violent rape is *reportable*. The man runs off into the night, the woman is picked up by the police, if she reports the rape at all, and she is generally taken to a hospital for examination. Sometimes she is treated like a culprit, though it has become common to treat her as the victim of a serious crime. Many cases of violent rape are not reported because the victim fears further abuse when she makes a public declaration of her already humiliating experience.

There are three more categories of rape, only two of which are reported to authorities or the public. The last kind of rape, the one whose existence is not even recognized today, is in fact the most common. It is reported here for the first time.

The second category of rape is the one in which a woman's submission is produced by intimidation or threats. There is little, if any, sign of violence and little, if any, court-admissible evidence. The reports of this kind of rape drop significantly because the victim fears, with some validity, that her story might not be believed. There is the case of "afterthought" rape, where a woman began a sexual act voluntarily, but at some point thereafter felt the need to allege rape. That allegation may or may not be totally valid. Every false accusation damns a hundred real victims by denying them credibility.

This question of legal reportability is crucial in determining the outcome of a nonviolent rape when it is reported. I recall a young woman who was brought to the emergency room of the hospital one night. She was shaken up but showed no signs of being harmed, though she was hysterical and vomited uncontrollably. She had been forced at knifepoint and under the threat of her life to have oral sex. She had not had intercourse at all. I remember a less than empathetic aide saying, "It's terrible, but at least she doesn't have to worry about getting pregnant, so everything will be all right."

The police were puzzled as to how to classify this woman's case because it was impossible to verify sperm in her vagina. They also admitted that it would be difficult to put together a case for assault and battery. Simply looking at this woman made it plain that there was nothing in the way of bruises, scratches, or torn clothing, which every policeman and doctor is taught to note carefully, that would substantiate a struggle. Everybody felt sorry for this young woman, but since she didn't fall into any neat legal category, a few motions were made but nothing was done.

Rape is more complex than most other crimes. It is not routinely reported when it occurs. Most victims are emotionally upset because the rape stripped them of their identity, dignity, and the right of personal decision. If they report this experience, they must publicly discuss it repeatedly, and this adds to their pain and humiliation. Simply put, a rape comes to the attention of the authorities and the public mainly when it can be substantiated in court. If there isn't any violence the rape is usually *unreportable*.

The experiences of women who have been raped do come to light in one place, however. This is my clinic, where individual counseling gives each woman a chance to discuss with a counselor, in complete confidentiality, why and how she became pregnant. Our counseling of patients indicates that there are two more categories of rape, and we have named them "social rape." Most startling, these are virtually unreportable forms of rape, they are significant contributors to unwanted pregnancy, and *the less reportable a rape, the more common it is in our society.*

Exactly what is social rape? We have defined it as any form of involuntary sexual activity that cannot be reported without destroying or seriously threatening a social unit, such as a marriage, family, or other significant relationship. There are two kinds of social rape, the first of which is sometimes revealed to a psychiatrist. The second is probably only discussed in an abortion clinic.

The first involves abnormal sexual encounters, such as intercourse between a parent and child, relations between relatives, certain instances of premarital sex, or sex with close friends of a family such as a long-time neighbor or baby-sitter. Consider crazy Uncle Bob, who was trusted enough to be left alone with his thirteen-year-old niece for an afternoon. Or Frank, who believes that Kathy's acceptance of his marriage proposal means that he can start their honeymoon right away. Or Jack, who's been attracted to his brother's wife for years. Or the tragedy of Laura, whose husband's best friend was home sick from work, came over for a cup of coffee and stayed for much more. In the confidence of communication with thousands of women, we have learned that these occurrences are present with an absolutely shocking degree of frequency.

Most of the time, this kind of rape involves long-standing relationships among relatives, friends, and fiancés, with whom sex was neither planned nor particularly wanted at the time, but occurred anyway. In these cases the men are not strangers. There isn't a physical attack, but intercourse is forced nonetheless. As these women generally describe it, making a public outcry and charging the man with rape would be totally destructive and unthinkable. Yet when an unwanted pregnancy occurs, the response of the last generation, a scandal or a shotgun marriage, is not wanted either. Marriage under these circumstances is felt to be an expansion of the tragedy.

The last and largest category of rape is the one that was least expected. This is social rape that occurs between a husband and wife *inside* of marriage. According to the law, sexual relations are a *right* of marriage. Even if reported, this form of rape would never be prosecuted.

It is difficult to pinpoint, with statistical accuracy, the number of problem marriages that persist simply because the people in them aren't ready to dissolve them. The large number of married women who need a pregnancy terminated indicates that many marriages are not strong enough to support an additional pregnancy. An unexpected pregnancy does not trigger a crisis for most happily married couples in their childbearing years. Pregnancy is, however, a very difficult situation for the woman who is utilizing all her resources to care for the children she has and still go through the agony of pretense to hold together the rest of her world.

A couple trapped in a problem marriage either may not engage in sex often, or sex may be sporadic and occur when least expected. Most of these women have a tendency to turn to some form of contraception other than birth control pills because they don't have sex with a moderate degree of frequency. Sheila describes what it is like: "We should have gotten a divorce years ago, but that's easier said than done. I told Jack never to come near me again and one time even scratched his face pretty badly with my nails. He beat me up when I scratched him, and he's right ... I won't ever do that again. The night this happened, he hadn't touched me in weeks. I was half asleep when I felt his hands on me. It scared me. When he's had a drink he can really make a mess. I didn't even have a chance to put in my diaphragm, and it was too late anyway. There wasn't any point in fighting him ... we have too many fights anyway. During the whole time, I just hoped and prayed that I wouldn't get pregnant. Well, so much for that. There was nothing else I could do."

This doesn't sound like the kind of rape the public reads about in newspapers. No body was found half buried in the woods. No woman was rushed by the police to a hospital emergency room to have her bruises bandaged and the medical tests for court made. This is social rape, and it is different. In a slowly dying but still existing marriage, sex can be claimed by the right of possession, with or without the wife's approval. This is not legally rape, but it is forced intercourse nonetheless. Coercion, fear, intimidation, or hopeless resignation play large parts in these rapes.

It is a striking paradox that the most common kinds of rape are the least reported for social or legal reasons. This is a shocking finding that both the public and professionals need to consider carefully. It is an overwhelming realization that the most common form of rape, and the one that produces a great number of unwanted pregnancies, is found in marriage itself.

Changing Attitudes of Women

Janice didn't think of herself as a feminist. She dressed, acted, and talked like most twenty-one-year-old college co-eds. She came to the clinic with a pregnancy that both she and her fiancé had attempted to avoid by using birth control pills. She had been scared by a number of confusing articles about the pill, and decided to play it safe by switching to foam. She used the foam properly, but as so many women learn, it isn't nearly as effective as the pill. In her next to last semester of college she became pregnant.

Finishing college was very important to Janice. As she put it, her degree was "a ticket into the real world." Except for her pregnancy, everything was headed in the right direction. She was a commercial art major and had an excellent portfolio from several summer jobs. By sending copies of it to New York, she had managed to obtain a job offer from an ad agency. Arthur, her fiancé, who was graduating at the same time, had gone to interviews and accepted an entry-level position with an investment house on Wall Street. Janice felt fortunate that her fiancé was pleased rather than threatened by her desire for a career.

Arthur accompanied her to the clinic. Though he felt no need to speak for her, he knew that his presence meant a lot, because this decision had been difficult for her. Janice said, "I feel that in a way I'm being selfish. I'm not against having a child, but it's just too early in my life."

Arthur agreed with her. "We do want children," he said, "but not now. We talked night after night about this. Neither of us are happy about it, but it would drastically change both our lives. We'd rather get established and then be able to have a family right."

This couple felt the need to explain themselves fully, and they gradually brought to light the depth of their concerns. "I know a lot of people wouldn't agree with my decision," Janice said, "and I wouldn't try to convince anyone else to think this way, but it's more than just putting a career in front of a family. I need to make my own place in the world and I don't want a family to be the only thing in my life. I want Art to love me and take care of me because he wants to, not because he has to."

"Explain why you feel that way," Arthur said. "You're not really selfish at all."

"I don't want to have the same kind of life my mother has had," Janice said. "She has all kinds of freedom and the house and all that, but she's had it. She's started seeing a psychiatrist from being nervous and upset. The worst part is that she doesn't have a good reason. At least a reason anyone understands. My father tells her to go and do anything she wants, just quit looking unhappy all the time.

"I think I know what Mom's problem is," Janice continued. "She doesn't feel her life is meaningful anymore. She had the chance, twenty years ago, to develop real interests, but it wasn't that important then. Maybe I had something to do with it when I came along. Anyway, she's great but she's in a mess, and I don't want to go down that road. That may sound like a terrible reason to have an abortion, but I mean it."

"Even without her mother's problems," Arthur said, "Jan is the kind of girl who has to make her own way. I agree with her about this pregnancy, because I don't want to see her lose the chance to have a life of her own."

An Identity of One's Own. Janice was talking about identity, her own identity. Without being an activist, she reflects the tide of changes that are altering the attitudes of many women and some men. She wants to be loved in all the ways that make her enjoy being a woman. She's not the least bit interested in competing against or dominating Arthur. But she wants an identity of her own in addition to being married to him.

In the past decade I've seen so many women in traditional roles who woke up wondering what significance their lives have had, other than taking care of a home and raising children. It's not that they were upset about doing either. Both, in fact, brought them pleasure, but they discovered they needed more. That extra something is the security of feeling that they are part of the entire world, not just a forgotten fixture in one corner of it. This awakening and these questions can be very upsetting, and they are known as an identity crisis.

Many women who have reached this stage in their lives have come to the clinic with an unexpected and, to them, totally catastrophic pregnancy. Their conflicts about being selfish and their need to establish new priorities for their lives are very intense, very difficult, and similar to the way Janice felt. The difference is that the feelings of middle-age women range from anxiety to panic when they realize that the time and energy to reorganize their lives are in short supply. Their task is considerably harder because they have greater obligations and fewer options.

Young women today have more options than they have ever had before. Janice struck me as having taken a considerable step forward from her mother's generation. She projected the positive attitude of being part of the world and actively reaching out to establish her own place in it. I've seen this vibrant determination in young women with greater and greater frequency. It is an unmistakable feeling that they have the right to their own identity, the right to a significant place in the world, and the right to determine their own destiny as they see fit.

The Supreme Court's decisions on abortion indicate the magnitude of this change. These court rulings are important in themselves, but their greatest significance is that they reflect an irrevocable change that has been building for many years.

The Emergence of Full Sexuality. The right to a complete, healthy sexuality is no more a new idea for a woman than the right to her own identity. Both have grown from marginal public awareness into the standard of what is normal in less than one generation's time.

The key to today's attitude about sexuality is that it is natural and good as long as it is natural and good. That statement may sound overly simplified, but it bears careful thought. It does not suggest promiscuity, which implies a series of meaningless relationships. It recognizes that sex may or may not be part of a special relationship, but when it is not it may sometimes be harmful. It rejects the idea that sex is sinful. It implies that its destructive consequences, including unwanted pregnancies, might be avoided. And it concludes that good sex is part of a normal life, because nature and God intended it to be there.

I've heard thoughts like these from women in their twenties, thirties, and forties. I've heard them from many teenage women who have accepted satisfying sex as part of their lives. Today, most women want to feel this way, as do most men. The main problem has been that the older a woman is, the more she's probably had to struggle with a massive amount of negative sexual conditioning, making complete fulfillment difficult for her.

The avoidance of unwanted pregnancies, through birth control, has made a large contribution to women's enjoyment of their full sexuality. I have been told quite a number of times that safe, legal abortion extends this inner freedom. For example, women know that if contraception fails and an unwanted pregnancy results, they still do not have to bear a child they do not want. Women can now realize the sexual side of themselves, as well as the possibilities of a social and economic identity, based on a wider range of values and goals than childbearing and homemaking.

Is Virginity Still Considered a Virtue? Gina was seventeen and had dated the same boy for two years. She wasn't impressed by her girlfriends' interest in sex. As long as she could remember, she had been taught that losing her virginity would mean losing her future husband's respect. This seemed reasonable, but from time to time she wondered whether she was missing something in the way of the famous sex drive she'd heard so much about.

The fact that Gina's boyfriend was very interested in sex seemed like a normal game that people play until they actually get married. This feeling was fine until their relationship went much deeper than dating and petting. The affection that she wanted to receive and then share had come to exceed the game of it all. She wanted to share herself.

Gina's attitude about sex had changed because she started thinking about love and not sex. As she described it, this went beyond all the teaching about virginity. It was much more than physical stimulation, and it no longer had anything to do with a calculated judgment of "respectability."

Gina overwhelmed me one day when she came into my private practice office for a checkup, six months after having received a prescription for birth control pills. She said, "You know, I've been close to my boyfriend for a long time and it really looks like we're going to get married after graduation. Everybody is happy for us."

"Congratulations, Gina," I said. "Just how is your relationship going? Do you have any questions?"

"Well, nobody knows we've been sleeping together, or at least I don't think they do. I've been bothered a little bit by it, you know, not being a virgin and all. I didn't want to talk about it to anyone but Jimmy, and, well, he just laughed. But I figured something out, and now I feel better."

"What's that, Gina?" I asked.

"I think virginity is okay because it shows somebody that he's extra special, like once-in-a-lifetime special, but all the lectures I've heard hardly talked about that at all. It was bad this and bad that and virginity was the only thing that mattered. I don't believe that anymore. I think it was just a form of birth control since nobody ever talked about the real stuff."

The lectures about the "bad this and bad that" of sex had certainly impressed Gina, but they wore thin because they lacked honesty in their intent. Much of that intent *was* to use abstinence from sex as a form of birth control. No one can say anything bad about recommending abstinence, but that recommendation becomes unrealistic once a relationship with a strong possibility of sexual activity begins. When the good and bad of the virginity argument begin to fail in practice, a serious discussion of real contraception must take place *before* the occurrence of an unwanted pregnancy.

Not all change is easy and not all change is good, but the discovery of mature sexuality is a healthy step for most young women. The bad effects of lectures on the importance of maintaining virginity have damaged many women of all ages. Even today, a large percentage of my patients are not really sure whether or not they should enjoy sex.

The interest of women of all ages in having their own sexual identities often parallels their reaching for identity in other areas of their lives. I've observed this interest expand with every passing year. All the changes, from testing virginity to a woman's establishing her own place in the world, will add depth, quality, and endurance to good relationships.

Marriage for Its Own Sake. In practice, the availability of legal abortion helps prevent marriages that would exist only because of an unwanted pregnancy. Its use also eliminates part of the myth that a bad marriage can be saved by an unexpected pregnancy.

It has been said that because of contraception and abortion, every pregnancy should be a wanted pregnancy. We have observed that a similar but bigger change is occurring in marriage for the same reasons. Today, the ideal is that *every marriage should be a wanted marriage*.

At the clinic we see daily that the time-honored, beautiful parts of marriage relationships have *not* changed. In fact, the best emotions found in marriage are desired more, and dead or dying marriages are tolerated less. The essence of a marriage is now a *continuing* love relationship between a woman and a man.

The Age of Contraception has given everyone a choice that never existed before. It has become easy to separate a deep emotional relationship from childbearing. This has been accompanied by the acceptance of divorce as an outlet from relationships that no longer work.

What we have learned is that marriage has not lost any of its positive meaning. If anything, it has gained greater meaning and dignity than ever before. This is the message that has made itself felt so strongly and repeatedly in discussions with thousands of women who have come to the clinic with their husbands or boyfriends. The relationship that many couples in past generations saw as a routine obligation has today become a valued option that is not taken lightly.

The Male and Unwanted Pregnancy

Men *are* deeply interested and very emotionally involved when a pregnancy touches their lives. This is not the popular understanding, however. Whenever men are discussed regarding pregnancy, the same reaction inevitably follows:

"Oh, yes. I guess men are interested, but I never thought about it much." This comment isn't foolish. It reveals that in pregnancies that are wanted, as well as pregnancies that present intolerable problems, the reactions of the man usually are considered as an afterthought, if they are considered at all.

Why should this be? Why do men seldom give the appearance of being deeply involved? Do they seem to be uninterested because they don't volunteer their thoughts or feelings easily or freely?

Dave, for example, stayed next to Christy all the way from the front door through the counseling room, and until she had to leave for the procedure. He was firm and quiet and knew that his presence was a source of strength for her. But he resisted talking much with the counselor, other than saying that he wanted to help Christy. Period. It was as if he were in a world in which he just didn't fit. He acted as if his job were to help, get out, and take care of her again once they were back home. He didn't think there was anything he could do for her as long as her pregnancy was still up in the air.

There is a large difference in the roles of men and women once a pregnancy has occurred. Although the man has taken a very active part in causing the pregnancy, his position is at least partly taken from him at the time pregnancy is confirmed. He can either support it or object to it, but he cannot make the final choice.

To a woman, pregnancy is a real, three-dimensional part of her body and mind. It alters the fabric of her whole future, regardless of whether she keeps it or ends it. No woman ever experiences the onset of pregnancy without this realization.

On the other hand, a man cannot have the same reaction throughout his whole body and mind. Pregnancy does not represent the same moment-to-moment reality and direct year-to-year continuity to a man that it does to a woman.

To the male, pregnancy is more of an idea than something real. He cannot touch it. He cannot feel it inside himself, or suffer his body's uncomfortable reactions to it. He can only imagine it. At most, he can visualize responsibility and appreciate the sensation of paternal feelings that nature has built into him to a relatively small degree compared to the woman. It isn't that he is insensitive or selfish. The combination of instinct and civilized training are limited in how far they can transmit into his sinews the feeling of what it is like to be pregnant.

The Prevalence of Machismo. Most men and women look forward to pregnancy as a beautiful miracle and a real blessing, when their relationship and conditions are favorable. But just as there are hundreds of circumstances which turn the prospect of a pregnancy into a nightmare for a woman, so the same numbers of circumstances apply to men.

But now comes the surprising part. We have been used to thinking that when an unwanted pregnancy occurs, it is always the man who wants to wash his hands of the whole matter and "get rid of the problem" as quickly as possible. We have imagined that it is the woman who finds herself in a relatively helpless position, more often than not wanting to keep her pregnancy in the face of overwhelming odds.

Frequently, just the reverse is true.

Lionel refused to come to the clinic at all. We learned about him from Wanda's explanation of his reactions. "Every time I went to talk about it," she said, "he'd get furious. He almost hit me yesterday. Stay home and have babies. That's all he wants. It's crazy. He doesn't even like the kids we have that much. I know what I've got to do, even if he's mad. I just can't understand him."

Contrary to the beliefs of all the old romantic novels, it is the woman of today who is apt to be the first to decide that she needs to limit and control what is happening to her. And it is the man who is more likely to want to have the pregnancy continue *whether or not* he intends to give the woman and her child any physical, financial, or emotional support.

This finding stopped us dead in our tracks and made us study it carefully. It occurred frequently with married men and their wives, as well as with single men and their girlfriends. It occurred with men of good income and education, as well as with men having less of both. Yet there was a difference that came to light in a review of our data and was verified by subsequent experience. The less the education and financial stability of the man involved, the more he tended to resist abortion, and the more he tended to leave the woman with the sole responsibility for continuing the pregnancy and raising the child. The pregnant woman is more than willing to discuss the problems she faces at home.

"What does your husband [or boyfriend] think of your pregnancy?" we ask in counseling.

"He thinks it is a problem. He really knows it's terrible."

"Why didn't he come with you to the clinic?"

"He doesn't like abortion. He wants me to have the baby. He's very firm about that."

"Is he going to take care of you or stick by you? Is he going to support you and the baby?"

The answers come back some yes, more maybe, and the greatest number, "probably not."

"But he still wants you to keep the pregnancy and take care of the baby yourself?"

"That's right," the woman usually answers.

We also wanted to find out why these women are pregnant in the first place. "Didn't you know about birth control?" we ask.

"Yes, I know about it, but he doesn't like it."

"Not even an IUD or the pill?"

"Not the pill or anything."

As this kind of discussion went on, the message that emerged was startling. "Is he making a good living or do you have problems supporting the children you have?"

"We have problems."

"But he wants you to have this pregnancy, too?"

"This and maybe more. But this is my pregnancy now and I can't go with it. I just can't and if he's mad, he's mad."

"You mean he wants you to keep having babies?"

"I don't think so, but it sure seems like it. It's something else, but he's funny about that."

Fortunately, relatively few men react like this, although we've discovered that many men on all economic and educational levels deeply resent losing control of their wives and girlfriends. This can cause difficulties if the woman decides to choose her own destiny against this kind of a man's wishes. Perhaps it is an inherent streak of what the Spanish call machismo. This is an attitude that combines the property right to control a woman, tribe survival instincts, and the need to frequently confirm virility. Sexually, it translates itself into sleeping with as many women as possible, fathering quite a few babies, but retaining the freedom to go or stay at will. This concept may be verbally rejected by the thoroughly socialized man in a jacket, tie, and vest, but it is a little gremlin found lurking behind a small corner of most male chromosomes.

In reality, almost all men know that this is not reasonable and works out to be somewhat ridiculous in practice. The image of a man wanting to be surrounded by a dozen small children whom he must raise has become rare if not nonexistent in this day and age.

The Frequency of Understanding. Just how often do men offer understanding to a woman who decides to have an abortion? Fortunately, in the greatest number of cases, men do have a depth of feeling, but in a practical sense they express it in a quiet abdication of control. Counselors and social workers like to say that "this male is supportive." What they are really saying is that he has found himself in a relatively helpless position, and he has taken the decent attitude of trying to make the whole thing as painless as possible for the woman.

At the clinic we encourage the father's participation in the counseling discussion of the best way to handle a problem pregnancy. With absolute regularity, we ask the man who does accompany the woman what he thinks about the pregnancy. Robert was a deliberate, thoughtful young man. His answer reflected thousands of similar responses. "Whatever she thinks is fine. I really want the best for her. We've talked about it a great deal and it's her decision. I'll help any way I can."

Both macho men and understanding men react to a very personal part of their lives that has been taken out of their control. Both types of men make the sometimes startling discovery that they can share sex but not a pregnancy, for which they have only an abstract idea of how to help a woman. The law reinforces this helpless position by saying that each woman may exercise her own judgment in this matter, regardless of the opinion of the man.

There is a fundamental difference between macho men and understanding men. The bottom line of the way a man reacts to an unwanted pregnancy is determined by whether he feels threatened by events beyond his control, or if he is strong enough to be able to really care for the welfare, feelings, and overall good of a woman, no matter what she chooses.

Antiabortion Tragedies

I'll never forget one of my clinic's first patients. Wendy's neat appearance—her attractive gray dress, silky long hair, and freshly scrubbed clean looks—didn't hide her feelings. She looked at me for a minute, as though to hang on to her courage, but her composure slipped. An involuntary sob escaped her lips. She raised her fist to her mouth and bit her knuckle.

This eighteen-year-old had two reasons to be on the verge of tears. The first was the problem that brought her to the clinic. The second was her mother, who at that moment was parading in front of the clinic, carrying a sign that read: Abortion Is Murder. Wendy had sneaked in the back door and her mother had no idea she was there.

It wasn't the sign or the demonstration that bothered Wendy. She was suffering because her mother's feelings were frozen in concrete. There could be no real communication about sex or abortion between them.

Wendy had grown up to be a sensitive and affectionate young woman. This outraged her mother, who insisted that she live by a narrow, rigid formula. Only fallen bridges remained. "If my mother sees me leave the clinic," Wendy said, "I might be disowned on the spot."

This young woman was deeply hurt by her mother's feelings, but in the end she didn't believe her decision was immoral or sinful. She was lucky. I could quote case after case of women who have been driven into depression or scarred emotionally because they accepted the label of being an immoral untouchable.

The burning brand of immorality is wielded frequently in the name of religious propriety. All religions plead for compassion. Most of the women I have seen subjected to painful guilt have been offered none.

I remember Agnes, a Catholic woman who faithfully followed the rhythm system through five pregnancies and could not bear another one. She suffered the unhappy fate of labeling herself an outcast and acting like one, even with people who did not know she had ended a pregnancy. It was months before this woman started treating herself decently, and it will be years before she recovers completely.

Many women are like Wendy and Agnes. They are surrounded by a constant barrage of propaganda against abortion. They are perfect candidates for an abortion, or even repeat abortions, since communication and accurate knowledge in this important area have been blocked out. Cause and effect are rarely mentioned, as are the real problems of a woman once she becomes pregnant.

The need for accurate information is multiplied dramatically by the event of pregnancy. By continuing to cut a woman off from real and authoritative communication at this time, antiabortionists help prevent her from making a decision based on *her* alternatives. Where problems are not individualized, the only benefits go to the self-righteous people who have inflated their own self-esteem.

Wendy and Agnes are only two drops of water in a deep river of socially reinforced guilt. Antiabortion proponents would have the public believe that they are only trying to prevent something, when in fact they are also causing and intensifying new tragedies. This is not known because most of the problems they cause are hidden in the silence of private guilt and suffering. Some of the other, more serious problems they cause are hidden by death.

Marie was thirty-seven years old. She had been a little overweight all her life, and in her twenties she was told that she had diabetes. Staying away from ice cream and cake when everyone else had a good time wasn't too bad.

Taking tablets later wasn't much worse. But after she married and had her first child a daily shot of insulin became a bother. With good medical care she was able to have three additional pregnancies. Marie was happy having children and raising them.

But each pregnancy did take its toll with flare-ups of the diabetic process. Her vision became a little worse. Her blood pressure climbed higher. Recurrent infections became a familiar part of her life. To make things worse, she became allergic to several of the antibiotics she needed, and others seemed to be losing effectiveness. After a while her doctor decided that her situation had turned into a long-term fight for survival. Anything straining her body's resources was best avoided, including pregnancy.

Before this couple had time to discuss the best form of contraception with their doctor, Marie became pregnant again.

When this woman first came to the clinic, signs of her being pulled in both directions were obvious. Her husband, on the other hand, was fuming. He was openly angry about the condescending comments of well-meaning friends who knew about Marie's need to terminate a pregnancy. They showed their sympathy by agreeing that it was a shame such a nice woman had to resort to what only trampy, bratty teenagers had anything to do with. The last straw, to him, was having a sign saying Murderer of Unwanted Babies shoved in her face while she was entering the clinic.

I could not tell Marie whether or not she would survive her pregnancy. I could only ask her to review what seemed most reasonable in light of her overall health and the best interests of her family. "I'm glad you're not pressuring me," she said. "I need more time to think about it."

Marie's thinking, I was told later, swung like a pendulum gone mad. One of her friends suggested that she give the other side a chance. Marie called the local pro-birth office and got a dose and a half of what she probably hoped to hear: how wonderful a good Christian woman she was for resisting the temptation of the easy, sinful way out. She was told not to worry about her family and health. Everyone knows that the Lord will provide. If He didn't want her to carry the pregnancy He would not have allowed it. "See your doctor and pray real hard. Don't fall into sin and everything will be just fine," she was told.

Everything was fine—until the eighth month of pregnancy. Marie developed an infection that involved not only her kidneys but her uterus as well. She went into premature labor and delivered an infant who soon died of respiratory distress. A week later she died as well, in acute kidney failure.

Cases like Marie's prove the mischief that can result from trying to impose the same formula on everyone's life. Even women like Wendy and Agnes were not helped by this formula.

The approach of the antiabortionists proves their lack of respect for individual judgment. True compassion for a woman's problems is based on respecting the judgment she brings to her own situation.

It is true that cases like Marie's do not occur often, as far as I know, but the problems of women like Wendy and Agnes are much more common. Even all the cases we know about at my clinic are only the tip of the iceberg, the greatest part of which lies invisible. But clues to its immensity surface often, when women explain in private counseling their reasons for coming to the clinic.

Lannie, a tearful twenty-seven-year-old, echoed the stories of hundreds of others when she said, "The last time I was pregnant I was talked into keeping it. I didn't want to, but everyone told me I was wrong. I kept it and it was a mistake. Now I'm being told the same thing again with this pregnancy. I want to listen, but I can't anymore. I feel trapped."

Beneath the clamoring righteousness there is a silent iceberg of suffering, and the antiabortionists refuse responsibility for the tragedies they cause.

The Surprisingly Wise Clergy: A Silent Majority?

The opening of my clinic in 1973 produced a rush of emotional responses from the community. They reached both extremes. The controversy lasted a full three weeks. When the storm subsided and we could finally devote total attention to the problems of our patients, the real caring and active support for women in need came from a group that surprised me very much—the clergy.

My education began with a phone call from a local minister. "He wants an appointment to talk to you," my secretary said. "You should see him. He's well known and respected."

The next day a bearded young man in a business suit was shown into my office. He appeared to be in his early thirties, was thin, and had black hair. His eyes were very intense, though his smile was delightful and easygoing. When he introduced himself he saw my reaction and said, "You look surprised."

"Frankly, I am," I said. "I expected someone in black with white hair. Forgive me if I'm out of line, but I think I'm pleased to meet you."

"Great," he said. "You don't look like a stuffed shirt either. Let me get to the point. In your TV interviews you spoke more about the patient than yourself or the clinic. I like that. I belong to a rather large group called the Concerned Clergy. It's nondenominational and it deals with helping people solve the real problems they have. Many of these problems have to do with catastrophic preg-

nancies. We make referrals, and if we are going to consider referring anyone to you, we need to know something
about you first."

I was speechless. "Do you realize that I'm guilty of
the same thing I accuse others of?" I asked him. "I've got
a stereotyped picture of what clergymen think, just as
other people have a stereotyped image of a woman who
needs an abortion. I definitely owe you an apology."

Until I met this minister I automatically assumed
that most clergymen are against abortion. Antiabortionists
often try to substantiate their views by claiming to have
a direct line to rightful thinking. I, like most people,
thought that anyone who interprets right and wrong for
other people would probably oppose abortion. Nothing is
further from the truth.

The years since that conversation have been a revela-
tion. I have found that I am in agreement with many of
the clergymen I meet, though we usually agree for different reasons.

Many ministers offer qualities of being available and
caring. Many of them have studied psychology, counseling,
or worked with mental health agencies. They have made
numerous quiet referrals to my clinic. Since they discuss
a woman's problems with her before she makes the decision even to visit a clinic, clergymen are often involved
from the beginning.

One couple, for instance, had a child who was born
with a physical defect. After they ran extensive tests, physicians told them it was genetic. But they could give no
guarantee of what would happen in a future pregnancy.
The most they could offer dealt with percentages. Though
a serious risk was present, this couple still conceived after
several years. Additional testing could offer no clear indication of the outcome of this new pregnancy. It was a very
distressed couple who visited their minister for help. He

assisted them in arriving at the decision they felt was best for them. Their case stands out because they needed much more than the review our counselors could offer.

Neither clergymen nor I "favor abortion," but we accept it as the last realistic solution to many unwanted pregnancies. Neither I as a doctor nor they as religious counselors receive comfort from assisting a woman in making the decision for abortion, regardless of her reasons. On the other hand, we know that the catch phrase "rape, incest, or the life of the mother" covers only a small percentage of the real problems that exist.

The majority of ministers in *all* religions agree that a woman who is forced, against her will, to go through pregnancy suffers just as much pain and anguish as the outrageous example of a woman who might be forced, against her will, to have an abortion. Consider that for a moment. It illustrates the kind of realistic, balanced thinking which, to my mind, the clergy have come to represent. They have felt the real concerns of women and their families. A large part of their calling and a deep test of their faith arises when they try to help solve these extremely difficult personal crises.

The clergy certainly has a spectrum of views on abortion. It has its share of dogmatic, inflexible table pounders, just as there are people like this in medicine, law, politics, or truck driving. In the end, most clergymen seem to have taken the position that the pregnant woman and her family must make their own decision. The most memorable statement of this concept was given before a large group from many professions. The speakers covered the abortion-related aspects of law, medicine, philosophy, and psychology, as well as religion. The pastor who addressed this meeting said, "Conscientiously relating to both God and people is my definition of love. When I help a woman reach her decision, I help her determine the best expression of her love for everyone in her life." It was interesting that at the end of the program the largest crowd, by far, collected around the man who spoke of love.

Other words that ministers frequently use are understanding and compassion. Most ministers describe their actions as searching for "what may be best," as opposed to "the lesser of two evils." Searching for what may be best helps a woman and her family create something positive, whether the decision leads to adoption, abortion, or continuing the pregnancy. These ministers could honestly claim that they offer love as the overriding determiner.

While most of the ministers I've spoken with have been Protestant, I have also talked with a considerable number of priests and rabbis. Formal discussion of abortion with the Catholic clergy is, however, limited in scope.

Informal discussions, on the other hand, have been lively and profound, and showed no lack of insight and personal interest. For instance, abortion has not always been condemned by Catholicism. It is condemned today, however, along with contraception, by the powers that be.

It surprised them that Catholic patients requesting abortion make up almost twice the percentage of Catholics in the general population, according to our statistics. This backs up the findings of various polls of the laity showing that the majority of Catholics favor safe, legal abortion. This is a profoundly difficult choice for Catholic women. I have seen many of them suffer deep guilt, possibly more than women of other religions, in spite of the fact that they had no realistic alternative.

Of the three major religions in America, Catholicism has expressed the greatest concern that answers be found that will eliminate abortion. The real issue is the *need* for abortion. In my opinion, this reflects the severe frustration the Catholic priests experience when they try to offer compassion to a woman who has a personal tragedy, but at the same time are unable to offer any means to prevent the tragedy. The net result is that many priests are not unfeeling, but they must remain unyielding.

I have also had the opportunity to speak with rabbis and Jews concerning the attitudes of the Jewish faith toward abortion. Orthodox rabbis are very similar to Christian fundamentalists. They interpret their religion to say that abortion is wrong. The majority of Jews are not of this persuasion. Religious personages do not speak for Judaism, because it is not governed by a hierarchy, as many Christian faiths are. In Judaism, each person has both the right and the responsibility for his or her own decisions.

Jews have survived by sheer determination, and this gives them the utmost reverence for life. They do not take life for granted, and place the quality of life ahead of its quantity. In general, the Jews I have spoken with do not consider abortion "good," even when there isn't any reasonable alternative. But they do recognize that an unwanted pregnancy can violate the quality of a woman's and her family's life, and they consider this worse. As a result, the great majority of Jews and their rabbis endorse legal abortion.

These discussions with clergymen have covered many controversial topics. Most discussions remained within the realm of interpretation. Some of the basic questions considered explain why this is so. They included: What is life? When is preventing a potential of life a blessing and when is it murder? When should any participant in an abortion feel guilty and when may he or she feel justified and elevated with the thought of having lessened a tragedy?

Numerous individual cases were brought up by all the participants, such as Ellen, a twenty-seven-year-old divorced woman who works full time and can barely support her six-year-old daughter and four-year-old son. What is a minister's responsibility when this woman says, "My boy-friend walked out when I told him I was pregnant. He wasn't much of a boyfriend anyway, but he was all I had. Now I don't know where to turn. Please help me decide what to do."

Opposite reactions can exist in the same clergyman at the same time. No single "answer" fits all situations, yet answers have to be found in simple enough terms to offer guidance for the women and families involved.

Out of this whole spectrum of communication, a clergyman's key question is often: When does a life become meaningful? I have heard men defend their views against birth control on the grounds that meaningful life consists of half a potential life. A single sperm or egg is enough to qualify. "Do you think that every time a pregnancy does not occur some kind of sin is committed?" is the unavoidable counterquestion. "No," is their answer, "not if it is the will of God. If it is the will of man then it is sinful. People are in sin anyway, and I am here to help them."

What is often taken to be the other extreme is the medical definition of viability. This is the accepted stage in pregnancy when there is a reasonable probability that a fetus might exist on its own outside its mother's body. This point of viability is judged to be approximately thirty-three weeks of gestation from the last menstrual period.

Most physicians, even those who have made a commitment to the need for abortion, have felt that this criterion is too extreme for performing the abortion procedure. Twenty to twenty-two weeks, or approximately halfway through a pregnancy, is the latest time at which a termination should be performed.

Sooner or later discussions come to the question of a soul. I have been asked the question "At what time in a pregnancy do you think a soul is present?"

I have had to back off from a direct answer to this question because I do not have a definition of soul. Everyone has the feeling that something like a soul should exist. Its ultimate meaning is that a human life is more than a collection of protoplasm, cells, and tissues. This is a reasonable thought, but doctors have not been able to show at what point in fetal development a soul comes into existence, because a medically applicable definition of the soul does not exist.

The one interesting medical concept of a soul that I have been able to offer results from studies of neurological development. Whatever a soul is, most people would tend to agree that it has to do with awareness beyond instinct or reflexes. Plants are not thought to have souls, yet even plants have simple reflexes such as growing toward the light. A one-celled animal, like an amoeba seen in a high school biology class, doesn't seem to qualify for possession of whatever a soul might be. Domestic animals like dogs and cats do seem to qualify. Their qualities are closer to the biblical concepts of selflessness and love than demonstrated by most humans.

The argument inevitably turns to the ability to think, as opposed to instinct or conditioning. It would seem that whatever a soul is, it is related to the ability to think.

In terms of human development, neurological research has shown that the brain begins functioning at about twenty-eight weeks. Since thinking is a function of the brain and since the soul seems to have something to do with thinking, then it might be reasonable to assume that a body and a soul may be capable of working together after about twenty-eight weeks.

I would never try to convince anyone of this particular premise, but if it should be absolutely necessary to structure a developmental formula for an unknown quantity using variable philosophies, the only constant being pregnancy, then whether this result is brilliant or absurd, it is nevertheless the best I can do.

Most clergymen avoided sweeping generalities based on their particular religious viewpoint. I had been preaching individualized medical and emotional evaluation of every woman's problems for quite some time. These discussions showed that the day-to-day practice of most clergymen places an equal emphasis on individualizing problems and solutions. There isn't any question that the basis for religious advice varies between groups, but the individual was usually considered no less than an individual who has unique problems and needs.

One final surprise took many discussions to verify and is of major importance. The opponents of legal abortion use the phrase "abortion on demand." This phrase gives the subtle impression of a haphazard, or thoughtless, decision. Clergymen do not believe that any woman takes the decision of abortion lightly. They know that, in reality, "abortion on demand" does not exist. The key point that astounded me was that this phrase symbolized, for many clergymen, a lack of compassion on the part of people who used it, even if they were of good intent. In many more ways than can be described, these men have repeatedly proved that they really care.

Rapidly Growing Public Involvement

With the passage of time—every day, month, and year—more and more people see for themselves the real needs and real problems of unwanted pregnancies in a very personal way. Up to 7 million people a year may be involved in the decision to have an abortion, assuming a conservative estimate of six other people directly touched by each unwanted pregnancy. One or more times a day in my clinic, a patient or a member of her family says that she or he always felt that any clinic that did what we do should not exist. As one grandmother put it, "I've picketed your clinic for years and I thought anyone who came here had no standards of their own." She hesitated, the tears welled up in her eyes, and she couldn't even finish what she had started to say. "Until... my granddaughter... well...thank you." The vast majority of parents, husbands, relatives, and friends of women who have an unwanted pregnancy are relieved to discover that emotional as well as medical care is an essential part of the treatment we provide.

The growing base of millions of personal experiences like these will continue to shape our nation's attitudes at large.

A historical parallel was the gradual realization that emotional illness is a treatable disease. This emotional need cried out for understanding of its depth, prevalence, and need for honest and dedicated treatment. Just as those who provide emotional care were able to shake off society's reluctance to admit the existence of emotional problems and bring those who needed help out of the cellars, so is quality abortion managing to lift public opinion out of the dark as well. Now it is fighting for recognition as a responsible and thoroughly competent medical and emotional service to which women can turn in good faith and with a clear conscience.

There is little question that one of the reasons for the current feverish campaigns of antiabortionists is the press of time. They are compelled to race against a swelling tide of direct public involvement, to suppress understanding, and to hope that compassion doesn't enter the minds and hearts of the millions of people who still don't know or who are still not sure. Once that happens, their appeal for public blindness will be lost forever.

IV

WHERE ARE WE GOING?

11

REPRODUCTIVE MEDICINE: THE SUCCESSOR TO OBSTETRICS AND GYNECOLOGY?

Five years ago we began with an idealistic approach to problems of abortion. At the moment when a woman faces the decision to keep or terminate a pregnancy, she must choose what her life is about and which direction she will steer it. Today, we have proven the value of highly personalized assistance that reflects our *patients'* feelings and *their* lives, instead of the opinions of the clinic or any one philosophy of life.

From this has come a greater ideal. The choice of family determination and self-identity by each woman, according to *her* needs and values, must be honored by the medical profession. In the field of abortion we have developed a comprehensive new standard of total personal understanding and assistance for *every* woman. If we agree that this kind of personalized care should be part of the procedure of an abortion, there is no reason for it to be less important in any other area. The time to propose a new approach to professional medical assistance to women and men has arrived and it could form a discipline that might be called reproductive medicine.

So many of the specialized reproductive needs of people are available only in scattered bits and pieces. There is dedication to emotional needs here, sexual needs there, physical problems of general medicine elsewhere. All of these serve specific purposes, but they have not been pulled together to best meet the emotional and physical problems affecting the chosen relationships of women and men.

The many medical procedures that involve the intimate parts of people's lives should be tailored to overall emotional as well as physical well-being. Understanding should be given to provide security in living with the affects of whatever needs to be done.

For example, every gynecologist has seen too many women who have had hysterectomies and after years of self-doubt have finally asked what could be done to re-establish their lost sexual interest.

"Wasn't it explained to you that your sexual drive would in no way be changed, except perhaps for the better, since whatever problems prompting the procedure would be eliminated?" the patient is asked.

"No, the doctor never went into that," is a standard reply. "I always thought that somehow the operation meant that I would be less of a woman."

"Do you feel like any less of a woman? Do you miss menstruating, for example?"

"No, of course I don't miss that. Sometimes I even feel like I'd like to let myself go."

"So what's the problem?"

"I guess I'm just not sure of what I'm supposed to feel and what I'm not."

The words in this kind of story certainly vary from patient to patient, but the message is the same and often repeated. A different kind of personal understanding and treatment is more essential in reproductive medicine than may be required in most other branches of medicine. A routine appendectomy or tonsillectomy, for example, has limited emotional involvement. The way the most intimate personal problems of women are solved may affect a woman for many years, and affect the other people in her family, according to the quality of care she receives.

In my opinion, the establishment of new centers of progressive women's medicine—based on a broader standard of professional care—is overdue. These should include medicine's latest technologies, such as genetic counseling, an ethical program of artificial insemination, and treatment of infertility, with no less care and attention to personal and family needs than we have developed in the field of abortion. It should also include advanced obstetrical techniques, directed at improving the safety and success of maintaining difficult pregnancies, as well as providing the best available emotional and medical treatment for both first- and second-trimester abortions, when and if needed.

Another prominent area of treatment should be sexual counseling. This now exists as a wasteland of rags and patches available only here and there, uneven in quality as well as in quantity. Where does a woman begin once she realizes that she has a problem that is progressively affecting herself, the man in her life, and perhaps her family as well? It is true that sexual problems may not be the primary factor in ending many marriages, but where they exist to a significant degree they certainly don't help. Does this woman go to a psychiatrist, a gynecologist, or an unlicensed sexual counselor? Is the emotional insecurity of something wrong in this area the cause or the effect of a basic difficulty which might be best helped by frank understanding, surgical correction, or a prolonged course of psychotherapy? In her own mind, a woman might ask, Where can I go to receive complete help with both the medical and emotional sides of my problem, without being labeled a neurotic or a foolish woman who is wasting a doctor's valuable time?

And how about the special problems relating to rape? How many general hospitals consider this emergency anything but an unpredictable nuisance to be dismissed by a few quick tests and quickly turned over to the police? The bewilderment, confusion, and shame that compels a woman who has been raped to run for cover demand a facility where all of her needs may be met with a minimum of fuss and a maximum of concern, understanding, and genuine assistance.

All these areas of medicine are subspecialties of gynecology and might be handled best under one roof. The fact that we are considering them as the basis for a new type of medical facility indicates that some women's criticisms of gynecology are accurate: They need help in more areas and ways than are presently available. The new concept of a specialty hospital offers a possible mature response by the medical profession to the changing needs of women. Like women themselves, medicine can break away from the ingrained attitudes that the main function of a woman is to have babies and that she is supposed to accept the idea of having all sorts of problems simply because she is a woman. These attitudes are deeply rooted in the thinking of our society and have served to prevent many women and many doctors from looking for solutions to them, or even admitting that millions of women suffer in silence.

Men may well be helped by this kind of specialized hospital, too. Believe it or not, a parallel set of deeply rooted attitudes is just as repressive to men. These are the beliefs that the main function of a man is to sire and support a family, that though he has the right to stress and personal problems, he is not supposed to admit them because this constitutes an admission of self-destructive weakness. Where does this man go for help, especially when his problems are deeply related to those of the woman in his life and his personal relationship with her? Psychiatry is not a universal answer. Neither are urology or gynecology, because they address only parts of the whole picture. Where might there be concerned medical and emotional help for the whole picture of changes that individuals and couples are experiencing in today's society? A concept of reproductive medicine that includes men as well as women is an entity of potentially enormously helpful dimensions.

What is the likelihood that this concept of medicine will turn into something real and three-dimensional in the near future? The straight answer is, "Not on a nationwide level." There is an excellent chance, however, that this will be pioneered in at least one or two specialized facilities somewhere in the country. From a medical, emotional, administrative, and, perhaps most important, financial survival viewpoint, all the pieces are here and, at least in my own mind, have come together to make an achievable whole. In presenting this abbreviated description of what gynecology might become, I make no pretense of having a sure formula to a medical heaven. It is only the start of a new attempt to present a serious medical response to changing personal and public needs.

APPENDICES

The appendices of this book offer an understanding of the changing status of abortion and an appreciation of new directions it may take in the near future. These directions involve law, medicine, legislation, and patient safety. The outcome will affect millions of lives each year.

Appendix A: *Briefing, Presidential Campaign '76*

During the Presidential campaign of 1976, abortion became a political issue wanted by neither side. Both parties felt obligated to take a position, and both reflected emotional opinions rather than factual information. Meaningless phrases like "abortion on demand" and references to who might or might not "favor abortion" were heard continuously. In all this oratory, two things became clear. The first was that no one demonstrated the benefit of having studied the subject, which might have been understandable because there was virtually no realistic information available other than propaganda. The second was that the forgotten person in all this sound and fury was the woman with the problem.

245

The following briefing was based on my studies prepared for this book. The Republicans took a stand to abolish all legalized abortion. The work was then offered to the Democratic campaign, and their health issues coordinator requested it on a priority basis. The Democrats won the election, but many outdated attitudes still remain to be changed. Abortion as a political issue is very much alive. You may well find this summary interesting and informative.

Briefing Paper on Abortion

1. What the decision to have an abortion is really like:

Pregnancies are received as a blessing most of the time. The American people strongly believe in the value of every life.

From the moment an unwanted or questionable pregnancy is discovered, the decision to have an abortion is an intense crisis for a wide spectrum of people. This decision is never taken lightly, regardless of the final choice. An abortion is *only* a last resort that is chosen when *no other* alternative is possible for the pregnant woman and her family. Under these circumstances, a safe, legal abortion is vastly preferable to an illegal abortion, which these women would be forced to obtain if abortion is made illegal.

2. Current public opinion on abortion:

A nationwide survey, commissioned by Knight Newspapers in February, 1976, at the height of the primary campaign of Ellen McCormack against abortion showed: 82 percent of Protestants and 98 percent of Jews agreed with the right to abortion. Seventy-six percent of Catholics agreed, 21 percent disagreed, and 3 percent said they did not know. Overall, 81 percent agreed. Other surveys have shown similar results.

Studies have shown that legalization has had the cardinal effect of permitting the woman who needs this procedure to obtain it openly, at a very reasonable cost, and under high standards of medical competency.

The legalization of abortion has *not* contributed to the need for abortion. Incidence is a function of need and *not* availability. There is relatively little difference in the statistical estimates in the incidence of illegal abortion as opposed to the incidence with legalization. Arguments to the contrary are based on negative emotionalism.

The pressures to make abortion a political issue represent the voices of a well-financed *small minority*. The majority of these people are Republicans—yet a Republican family rushes their pregnant teenage daughter to my clinic for an abortion just as fast as a Democrat's family. We also see a steady trickle of Right-to-Life parents as the problem touches them directly.

3. What is the statistical need for abortion?

The public's requirements for this procedure are 10,000 per million per year. A cross section of all the population is represented with one notable exception. There is a disproportionately *higher* incidence of Catholic women who have abortions. Thirty-eight percent of all the patients seen in my clinic gave their religion as Catholic, whereas the general population of Central Florida reflects a base of approximately 22 percent.

AGE:

19.0% Under 18	(Central Florida Statistics)
54.6% 18–24	
15.1% 25–30	
10.5% 31–40	
1.3% Over 40	

The majority of married patients are twenty-five and over. The majority of single patients are below the age of twenty-four. Of the single patients, 85 percent report a one-to-one relationship of long standing, with contemplation of marriage, thereby negating the implication that promiscuity is a significant cause of unwanted pregnancy.

RACE:
    82.0% White   (Central Florida Statistics)
    17.5% Black
    0.3% Other

Initially, only the black upper and middle classes applied for abortions. With dissemination of information, the figures advanced to those of the general population percentage. Blacks and whites have the same rate of need for abortion. The figures are not disproportionately higher for either group.

There is a greater resistance to abortion on the part of the black male than the white, despite no increased demonstration of financial or marital support. The black male's concern is a synthesis of pride in producing the pregnancy and a suspicion that abortion is a form of genocide against blacks.

RELIGION:
    55.0% Protestant   (Central Florida Statistics)
    38.0% Catholic
    2.0% Jewish
    4.8% Other or No Religion Given

The disproportionate percentage of Catholic women is attributable to conditioning against contraception and the equation of contraception with promiscuity ("I'm not *that* kind of woman.")

INDICATED REASONS FOR HAVING AN ABORTION:
    73.7% Social   (Central Florida Statistics)
    21.8% Economic (financial hardship)
    4.1% Physical (health of the mother)
    0.3% Nonphysical

Social pressures include rape, emotional stress, teenagers who haven't the maturity to become parents (as young as age nine), etc. Economic indications rose to a short-lived peak of 30 percent during the Arab oil embargo, reflecting financial hardships and insecurities.

REFERRAL:

    36.1% Physicians   (Central Florida Statistics)
    12.6% Health Departments
     8.6% Agencies
    42.8% Miscellaneous

Miscellaneous referral includes a surprisingly significant number of clergymen. This professional group is the *most* concerned and supportive of all the various professionals in the field. Physician referral has shown a steady increase since legalization, reflecting the medical community's increasing acceptance of abortion.

4. What kinds of people have abortions?

People who recognize the need for abortion identify with women who have problem pregnancies. Examples of such women are one of age nine, who is still a little girl; age thirteen, made pregnant by experimenting with her twelve-year-old brother; age sixteen and so conditioned against sex that she couldn't admit a sexual relation; age nineteen and not ready to have a child; age twenty with an engagement ring and a year short of her college degree; age twenty-one and not ready for marriage; age twenty-three and told by her physician she could never get pregnant because of a tipped uterus; age twenty-four and abandoned by her boyfriend when she became pregnant; age twenty-seven and the mother of two who was deserted by a husband bored with family life; age thirty and broke off with her boyfriend when he showed no support for her pregnancy; age thirty-four and told by her boyfriend of a nonexisting vasectomy; age forty-one and raped by an overly friendly friend of the family; age forty-four and just learned she has breast cancer; age forty-nine and missed a few periods and assumed she was safely into menopause; and age fifty-three and scared of the certain negative reaction of her husband, children, and grandchildren.

In short, an unwanted pregnancy can occur in almost every family in every social and economic area of society.

5. Who favors abortion?

Nobody *favors* abortion, but the great majority of people have come to recognize the need for this procedure. An extremely large number of religious groups and professional associations have endorsed the need for the procedure on an individual basis. A list is enclosed at the end of this briefing.

6. Why do some people oppose legal abortion?

There are essentially three groups of people who are against legalization. The first are those who are opposed on religious grounds. This includes the minority of Protestant religions and the minority of the Catholics, as demonstrated by the previously quoted survey.

Second are those who cannot identify with a woman in distress.

Third are those who visualize the image of elevating their personal moral stature before others and to themselves.

The totality of these people are in the minority, though the few who are organized are well financed and vociferous.

7. What are the medical abortion procedures?

First trimester (first twelve weeks of pregnancy): During this period the procedure utilizes the suction evacuation of the uterus. It is called suction curettage and, according to public health figures, carries less mortality and morbidity than a normal pregnancy carried to term, or even a tonsillectomy.

Second trimester (second twelve weeks of pregnancy): This is a more complex procedure that involves injecting medication into the uterus, leading to a miniature labor.

The first-trimester procedure can be carried out in a clinic or a doctor's office. The second-trimester procedure is performed in a hospital. The lack of availability of this second-trimester procedure (many hospitals refuse to perform it) has caused untold emotional and financial hardship to many women in desperate need. In many parts of the country they must travel hundreds of miles for this procedure.

With adequate counseling and proper medical care,

there need be no significant adverse effects regarding future pregnancies or emotional scars to the patient from either of these procedures.

The beginning of the third trimester is the time of potential fetal viability, and no doctor has any interest in terminating a pregnancy beyond this point.

I am an advocate of firm state regulation of medical abortion practices, covering both the emotional and physical welfare of the patient. To my surprise, I have met great resistance in the adoption of high quality public health guidelines.

8. Government deficits:

Whether from the lack of birth control information or contraception in public health clinics, or from public fright caused by the unbalanced release of information on birth control safety by the FDA, the net result is that the Republicans have failed to address themselves to eliminating at the very least some of the causes of unwanted pregnancy—which *can* be eliminated.

Decrease of funding for family services and family planning is another deficit.

This is a serious failure of leadership because prevention is always better than treating a problem after it has occurred. Denying access to abortion or claiming that the need for abortion should not exist, while failing to prevent at least some of the causes of unwanted pregnancies, is hypocritical.

The Republican support of a ban on abortion is also a serious contradiction in their basic "anti–big government" campaign posture. Banning abortion removes an individual's right to choose. It expands the power of the government at the same time that they campaign against this very power over people's lives.

9. What the Carter administration can do to lessen the need for abortion:

There are preventable causes of unwanted pregnancies, and they are being studied intensively by physicians like myself.

A commission should be appointed to correlate information gathered by research-oriented physicians and organizations active in this field. This information can be disseminated to the public, clinical physicians, public health departments, and social agencies for realistic approaches to the problems.

The FDA must continue to advise the medical profession and the public on its evaluation of the safety of contraceptive drugs and devices. The Carter administration should direct this agency to present that information with sufficient perspective so that physicians and patients do not abandon beneficial contraceptives because of fear alone. There have been far too many instances of one minor finding, not even fully substantiated, resulting in a flood of women arriving at the clinic with unwanted pregnancies.

Restoration of funding for family services and planning is important. It can help strengthen a family unit in which every pregnancy is a wanted pregnancy. Further benefits should include decreasing the incidence of child abuse, runaways, premature sexual encounters, and abandonment of education with subsequent refuge in the relief rolls and juvenile crime.

There should be the kind of sex education in the schools that the public will want. This is education *with the participation of parents* so that parents do not have to fear loss of direct input into the thinking and values of their children.

The Carter administration should defend Medicaid support for family services, family planning, and abortion. Ending this funding discriminates against the poor who often need these services desperately. Before and after legalization, those who could afford it always had these services available.

10. Answers to the questions I am most often asked about abortion:

Permit me to offer responses I have made to the most negative and severely antagonistic questions to my posture on every woman's right to choose whether or not to continue a pregnancy.

a. *"Do you favor abortion on demand?"*

There isn't any such thing as abortion on demand. That phrase implies a frivolous request. It implies that a woman would seek an abortion just because it is available. This is utter nonsense. No woman takes this decision lightly and no physician accepts it lightly, regardless of the liberality of his feelings. Requests for this procedure are made only as a last resort, reflecting a deep tragedy in a woman's personal life.

b. *"When and what is life?"*

Life is medically accepted as beginning at the point of the ability for survival. In obstetrics that point occurs at approximately thirty-three weeks of gestation. From the standpoint of abortion, no responsible physician to my knowledge has the least interest in terminating a pregnancy beyond twenty-two to twenty-four weeks, the upper limit of the second trimester.

c. *"When does the fetus have a soul?"*

Discussion of a soul is difficult because a definition of a soul is almost impossible to agree upon. The most realistic medical answer to this philosophical question is the equation of a soul with twenty-eight weeks, at which time it is estimated that the brain is capable of functioning.

d. *"How can anyone stop a life and still have Christian love?"*

Love is a question of compassion. Many decisions are extremely difficult, but must be made. The decision to extend the compassion of abortion to a pregnant woman with problems and a desire to terminate her pregnancy is the only valid answer to that question.

e. *"What do you say to pictures of this fetus?"*

The pictures are significant and do make us feel awe for the potential of life. But the pictures of women in tragedy also come to mind, showing thirteen-year-old girls with pregnancy, victims of rape, and the vast multitude of women who simply cannot cope with a pregnancy for a thousand individual reasons. It is a question of identification. I feel for the woman with a tragic pregnancy and have dedicated myself to helping her.

f. *"Would you let your wife or daughter have an abortion?"*

My family and I feel fortunate and truly blessed because each pregnancy represented a gift of joy. The need has not existed, I am thankful to say. This realization does not prevent me from recognizing that many other women and many other families may not always be so fortunate.

g. *"How can a doctor and patient alone make this great decision?"*

Only the woman and her doctor can come to appreciate the many personal aspects of her life, training, and relationships with the rest of the world and evaluate this most personal decision. No subject, especially pregnancy, should ever be decided on the basis of formula.

h. *"What do you think of the Right to Life?"*

I agree with the reverence for life. I also respect the quality of life that already exists in the form of a real woman with real problems, a real family, and the real right to determine her own destiny as much as possible.

i. *"How about the Supreme Court's decision that parents have no legal control over their daughters?"*

The Supreme Court's decision does not in any way decrease the influence of parents on their child's maturity so long as that influence does in fact exist. In reality, the matter has greater effect on the young women in whom that influence has long since disappeared. The most striking day-to-day effect seen turns out to be the opposite of what you'd expect. This occurs in the instance of the pregnant child of ages ten to thirteen with no concept of the meaning of parenthood who wants to have and play with her baby ... and the parents are powerless to take what they think may be her best course of action. Once again, the answer lies not in legal interpretation so much as in the strength of the family unit.

Appendix B: *Model State Laws to Assure Quality Abortion: A Three-year Fight in Florida*

The 1973 Supreme Court ruling struck down most but not all state power to regulate abortions. It left the states with the right to "regulate the abortion procedure in ways that are reasonably related to maternal health" in the second trimester. There have been many attempts to translate this right into statutes in various legislatures. These attempts have been muddled by a scramble of personalized opinion on the part of both anti- and pro-abortionists, each of whom is attempting to exert his or her own influence.

The people against abortion have tried all kinds of devices to restrict availability and accessibility of this service, and at several points they have succeeded. Their most notable success was the Hyde Amendment, in which the 1976 U.S. Congress first restricted Medicaid funds for payment of abortions for poor women who may well have the most need for it.

On the other side of the fence, outspoken groups have opposed every kind of regulatory legislation with the fear that any regulation would lead to total regulation and that total regulation would produce lack of availability.

The controversy has roared back and forth, with neither side winning the war. The result is that the advocates of both extremes are backing into each other by coming full circle in the impact of their positions. Each side has become so involved with its own mad scramble to be heard that it has forgotten the welfare and safety of the patient.

The plight of the woman in need is that she is turned into a forgotten victim who may be hurt by each side's total commitment to an opinion. Both total restriction and total abandon lead to incompetency and inadequacy of safe abortions. Both groups are perilously close in their net results, the butchery of women in need.

This situation became clear to me three years ago and I began fighting for state legislation that empowers my state's health department to establish at least minimal standards of medical safety for the performance of these procedures. This must and can be done in such a way as to avoid any harassment or restriction of access to abortion, so long as that access does not constitute a wanton disregard of accepted medical standards of safety.

In taking this position I lost the support of both the antiabortion and the proabortion groups. They are not my concern. I have made my plea to legislators, health officials, and others on the grounds of patient safety. It would be an overwhelming tragedy to see the benefits of legal abortion degenerate to the point where the quality of care may not be much different from what it was in the horrible days before legalization.

Model Law

TO: Committees on Health, Florida Legislature

SUBJECT: Request for filing a bill for ensuring minimal health standards through licensure of abortions past first trimester.

NEED FOR LEGISLATION: Pursuant to Supreme Court decisions on abortion of January 1973, Florida Statutes 458.22 relating to restrictions is interpreted as being unconstitutional by Robert L. Shevin, Attorney General, in his widely distributed analysis of 2 Feb. 73. This statute has never been stricken. It has simply been ignored and the state has no viable statute.

Such a statute is needed for instances from and after the first trimester in the name of protection of maternal safety. Current threats of wholesale provision of second trimester procedures free of any medical safeguards on outpatient bases brings the issue to immediate relevance. For better or worse, it is conceded that first-trimester procedures may not be regulated. Procedures thereafter may be and should be through statute restricting performance to facilities properly licensed and therefore subject to compliance with health standards as may be delineated by Florida Department of Health and Rehabilitative Services.

Relevant Supreme Court References Decided January 22, 1973:

A. JANE *ROE* v HENRY *WADE* (410 US 113)

1. The state has a legitimate interest in seeing to it that abortion, like any other medical procedure, is performed under circumstances that ensure maximum safety for the patient.

2. The state's legitimate interest in seeing to it that abortions are performed under circumstances that ensure maximum safety for patients extends to the performing physician and his staff, to the facilities involved, to the availability of aftercare, and to adequate provision for any complication or emergency that might arise.

3. From and after the end of the first trimester of pregnancy, a state may regulate the abortion procedure to the extent that the regulaion reasonably relates to the preservation and protection of maternal health.

4. A state statute which restricts legal abortions to those "procured or attempted by medical advice for the purpose of saving the life of the mother" sweeps too broadly to withstand constitutional attack because it makes no distinctions between abortions performed early in pregnancy and those performed later, and because it limits the legal justification for the procedure to a single reason, namely, "saving" the mother's life.

B. MARY *DOE* v ARTHUR K. *BOLTON* (410 US 179)

1. A state may adopt standards for licensing all facilities where abortions, from and after the end of the first trimester, may or must be performed, so long as those standards are legitimately related to the objective the state seeks to accom-

plish, though such facilities may not be limited to licensed hospitals only.

2. A state may not require that abortions, prior to the end of the first trimester, be performed only in hospitals.

Request for Filing of Bill Stating That:

Be It Enacted by the Legislature of the State of Florida:
458.22 Termination of Pregnancies

1. DEFINITIONS.—As used in this section, unless the context clearly requires otherwise:

a. "Physician" means a doctor of medicine or osteopathic medicine licensed by the state under chapter 458 or chapter 459 or a physician practicing medicine or osteopathy in the employment of the United States or this state.

b. "Approved facility" means a hospital or medical facility licensed by the Department of Health and Rehabilitative Services pursuant to rules and regulations adopted for that purpose regarding performance of abortion, provided such rules and regulations shall require regular evaluation and review procedures, and reasonably relate to the preservation and protection of maternal health.

2. TERMINATION OF PREGNANCY.—For the purpose of the preservation and protection of maternal health, it shall be unlawful to terminate the pregnancy of a human being unless the pregnancy is terminated in an approved facility by a physician. In any instance of termination from and after the end of the first trimester of pregnancy, termination must be performed in a licensed hospital or only in a facility specifically approved for that purpose.

3. WRITINGS REQUIRED.—The written request and consent of the pregnant woman or that of court appointed guardian in cases of mental incompetency shall be obtained by the attending physicians.

4. Reporting procedure.—

a. The director of any medical facility in which a pregnancy is terminated pursuant to this section shall maintain a record of such procedures. Such record shall include the date the procedure was performed, the reason for same, and the period of gestation at the time the procedure was performed. A copy of such record shall be filed with the department of health and rehabilitative services, which shall be responsible for keeping such records in a central place from which statistical data and analysis can be made.

b. Records maintained by an approved facility pursuant to this section shall be privileged information and deemed to be a confidential record and shall not be revealed except upon the order of a court of competent jurisdiction in a civil or criminal proceeding.

c. No records required under this section shall contain information which would permit the identification of any person whose pregnancy is terminated pursuant to this section.

5. Right of refusal.—Nothing in this section shall require any hospital or any person to participate in the termination of a pregnancy, nor shall any hospital or any person be liable for such refusal. No person who is a member of, or associated with, the staff of a hospital nor any employee of a hospital or physician in which or by whom the termination of a pregnancy has been authorized or performed, who shall state an objection to such procedure on moral or religious grounds, shall be required to participate in the procedure which will result in the termination of pregnancy. The refusal of any such person or employee to participate shall not form the basis for any disciplinary or other recriminatory action against such person.

6. Penalties.—

a. Any person who performs, or participates in, the termination of a pregnancy in violation of the requirements in subsection (2) of this section which does not result in the death of the woman shall be guilty of a felony of the second degree, punishable as provided in 775.082, 775.083 or 775.084.

b. Any person who performs, or participates in, the termination of a pregnancy in violation of the requirements in subsection (2) of this section which results in the death of the woman shall be guilty of a felony of the second degree, punishable as provided in 775.082, 775.083 or 775.084.

    c. Any person who violates any provision of subsections (3) or (4) of this section shall be guilty of a misdemeanor of the first degree, punishable as provided in 775.082 or 775.083.

This act shall take effect July 1, 1977.

Appendix C: *Model Guidelines for First-trimester Abortion Procedures*

The Supreme Court said that the state has a legitimate interest in seeing to it that abortion, like any other medical procedure, is performed under circumstances that ensure maximum safety for the patient. It then spoke about regulation only from and after the first trimester.

    That position seems to speak against statutes restricting availability of first-trimester procedures, but appears to create no prohibition against publishing health department guidelines for minimal standards of safety. The net result of this position should be the same as any other medical procedure, such as tonsillectomy or appendectomy. Granted, those procedures have not carried the emotional charge that has accompanied the evolution of abortion. Nevertheless, if patients undergoing tonsillectomy and appendectomy enjoy the security of certain health standards, then patients requiring abortion deserve no less.

    The strength of these guidelines would not necessarily lie in the ability to grant or withhold licensure. That ability could automatically carry the power to close any clinic or medical office performing these procedures. There is a justified fear that this power might be used dictatorially by any director of health who might place his own personal persuasion above the obligation of public trust. An outrageous example of this possibility occurred in the early days of the Carter administration when Califano, the Secretary of Health,

Education and Welfare, announced his position as an anti-abortionist and stated that he would do all in his power to suppress accessibility for the procedure. The existence of this kind of tyranny could weigh the balance against licensure of legitimate first-trimester facilities.

On the other hand, the effects of published guidelines that are reasonable and express the sincere concern of the state for the needs of all its people would have strength in a medico-legal sense. The facility providing first-trimester abortion in a haphazard fashion or one with less than total concern for the welfare of the patient would be liable to the patient herself. That seems eminently fair. The level of that concern could be and should be reflected in health department guidelines.

To assure that those guidelines are objective and reasonable, they should carry the endorsement of authorities directly concerned with specific procedures and potential problems. These authorities should be at the very least statewide societies of obstetricians and gynecologists together with the opinions of professors of gynecology at medical school teaching centers. They should also reflect the input of physicians directing clinics providing public access to the procedures themselves. With this view in mind the following recommendation of the Florida Obstetrical and Gynecological Society is presented:

Recommendations of the Florida Obstetrical and Gynecological Society Pertaining to Approved Facilities Conducting Terminations of Pregnancy

I. DEFINITION

1. Termination of pregnancy: Any act or procedure, medical or surgical, performed by a physician under the provisions of Chapter 72-196 Laws of Florida for the purposes of interrupting a pregnancy.

2. Approved facility: Hospitals licensed by the Division of Health under Chapter 395, Florida Statutes, and outpatient facilities meeting the requirements delineated hereunder.

II. FACILITY ADMINISTRATION

1. Each facility shall be designated by a distinctive name and the name shall not be changed without obtaining proper registration with the State.

2. The following information shall be required on the premises:

   (a) Identification of ownership and responsible authority.
   (b) Descriptive plan including physical plant.
   (c) Documentation of registration with the State as a medical office, clinic, hospital, etc.
   (d) Indication of nearby hospital privileges on the part of the medical staff; or arrangements for hospital admission in case of an emergency; or transfer agreements between the facility and a nearby hospital.
   (e) Indication of real and anticipated community need based upon population, open for review by the Division of Health at all times. Disclosure to area-wide Health Planning Councils as to community need should also be part of the facility's documentation.

3. A roster of Florida licensed physicians, registered nurses, licensed practical nurses, and medical technicians shall be kept together with current registration numbers.

4. A licensed physician, registered nurse, and medical technician shall be present at the facility no less than five days of each week, not counting holidays.

5. The facility shall maintain twenty-four-hour, seven-day-per-week, emergency call service so that no patient may ever experience difficulty in obtaining contact and assistance from the facility in the event of emergency.

6. It is mandatory that the operating physician be skilled in the necessary gynecological procedures to be performed. It would be preferable that he be certified by the American Board of Obstetrics and Gynecology.

7. Discharge of patient from the facility shall be made

only by an attending physician when in his judgment the patient may be released without jeopardizing her health and safety. If for whatever reason it is considered by the attending physician unsafe to release the patient, and an overnight stay is necessary, she shall be transferred to a licensed hospital for such care as may be required.

8. The facility shall establish a program to insure post-termination follow-up for each individual treated, consisting of examination and appropriate treatment.

9. The facility will be used for first-trimester pregnancies only. All second-trimester pregnancies shall be terminated in a licensed hospital facility.

III. COUNSELING

1. The objectives of counseling include:
   (a) Alternative counseling should be provided.
   (b) Direction to postabortal follow-up and/or therapy.
   (c) Efforts concerning prevention of the necessity for abortion from whatever causes.
   (d) Familiarization with forms of contraception if indicated.
   (e) Individual attention as opposed to group guidance.

IV. USE OF ADVERTISING

No person, association, co-partnership, corporation, or facility shall advertise to the general public its being approved or licensed for the purpose of performing procedures resulting in termination of pregnancy.

V. SURGICAL SERVICES

Facilities not licensed as hospitals and those licensed hospitals not regularly affording obstetrical, gynecological, or surgical services shall provide facilities consistent with the needs of termination of pregnancy procedures. As a minimum they shall include:

1. Surgical operating rooms having usable floor space of

at least ninety square feet, containing adequate operating facilities with ready access to suction, oxygen, defibrillator, resuscitator, intravenous supplies, and instrument stands.

2. Adequate areas for sterilization of equipment and storage of medical and surgical supplies.

3. One or more recovery beds or lounges, not to exceed five per operating room. A minimum of one toilet facility per six recovery areas shall be provided for the use of patients. The recovery room areas shall have ready access to the above emergency supplies and equipment.

4. Flammable anesthesia is prohibited in facilities unless the operating rooms and supporting facilities meet the requirements of NFPA 56A Standards for the Use of Inhalation Anaesthetics (1970) for anesthetizing locations. If used in outpatient facilities, nonflammable general anesthetics should be employed by a licensed nurse-anesthetist or anesthesiologist.

VI. MEDICAL RECORDS

A medical record with appropriate history, physical exam, emotional evaluation, and laboratory results as well as notes of the procedure and any follow-up visits shall be kept on each patient.

VII. LABORATORY SERVICES AND FACILITIES

1. Diagnosis of pregnancy and physical sizing of the uterus shall be made by examination prior to each procedure. In case of question, pregnancy test may be used, notwithstanding recognition that neither exam nor test are foolproof in early gestation.

2. A licensed medical technician shall be on duty in the facility no less than five days of each working week.

3. A gross and microscopic identification of products of conception shall be performed.

4. Preoperative laboratory data shall include urinalysis, hemoglobin, serology, and Rh factor. Immune globulin shall be available to Rh-negative patients who are candidates.

VIII. SANITATION, HOUSEKEEPING, AND MAINTENANCE

Each facility in which termination of pregnancy procedures are performed shall maintain the total environment in a clean, safe condition, and in good repair. Contaminated wastes, linens, and supplies shall be kept and transported in covered containers specifically for this purpose.

> Approved by the Executive Board and the membership on 5/7/76
>
> William H. Kirkley, M.D.
> President Florida Obstetric and
> Gynecologic Society

Appendix D: *Expert Testimony by Samuel J. Barr, M.D., Before the U.S. House of Representatives, Committee on Ways and Means on National Health Insurance: The Role of Government in Abortion and Contraception*

The prime targets of the antiabortion groups are the weakest and least influential women and families of this country, the poor who require government health assistance. On a larger scale, national health insurance has been studied and debated for many, many years in efforts to find a plan that would be beneficial to the people and acceptable to the providers of health care in such a manner so as not to bankrupt the federal treasury. This area has been the object of the lobbying attack of the antiabortionists for some time. Their motivation is simple. If they can force their views into this legislation, then with one stroke they can eliminate access to needed abortion without ever having to take their case to the public. There are so very few voices to speak for the majority of real people with real problems. Even fewer opportunities are available to the average person or even the concerned physician. I had one such opportunity in June of 1974. I am presenting my contribution to the testimony because the issue is still to be decided and will be in debate and under attack for many years to come, regardless of the initial form of national health insurance that may be passed.

Statement of Samuel J. Barr, M.D., EPOC Clinic, Winter Park, Fla.

DR. BARR. *Thank you, sir. I am Dr. Samuel Barr. I am a gynecologist and obstetrician in private practice. I also direct a clinic that is dedicated to family planning and abortion in light of recognizing some of the needs in this area.*

I would like to thank you for the chance to speak today because of the fact that legislation which will affect all aspects of medical treatment the area of abortion and contraception and family planning has been under attack very vigorously, and I am sure that this attack will be carried here as well, by certain groups primarily with religious motivation, in the overall effort to have the Government disallow funding for these services.

These services may be unpopular, but the point I would like to leave with you gentlemen today is that they are quite, quite important. There are several issues involved. The first is that of the Congress deciding what medical procedures and what problems may or may not be treated. I don't think—I certainly hope it is not the intent of Congress to do this. But with national health insurance, which will certainly supersede all other forms of assistance, if the Congress should be convinced of disallowing funding for any aspect of medical care, that will in effect prohibit all patients needing such care from getting it.

The second point is that of abortion, per se, and the only one thought that I hope to leave with you today on this complex topic is that for patients requiring such service it is an overwhelming necessity. I will ask you to accept that. I can give you many, many, many examples of why this is so, and I would be happy to do so if you would like to question me further on that point.

It is a necessity and one which no one, neither patients nor physician nor clergymen nor social workers take lightly. It is a topic of great moment, but one of necessity that is unquestionably present.

The third point—and there are only four that I would like to make—is that with the political pressures being applied against this area of the practice of medicine—I think that the point must be made of the importance of keeping separate one group's philosophies or religious convictions from legislation that affects all of the country. This precedent, as you know better than I, goes back all the way from separation of church and State to antitrust legislation.

The last issue is that of economics, which must come into any discussion. It is simply the recognition of the realistic sound economics of not forcing unwanted pregnancy, or pregnancy which cannot be adequately handled by the indigent, or anyone else for that matter.

The case in point arose in the Senate recently in which an amendment was added to the Social Security Act, specifically prohibiting medicaid funding for anything to do with the area of reproductive medicine. This I think for the reasons I suggested is a rather frightening prospect from many aspects.

I would like to make a few short recommendations, and the first is that the Congress not disallow medical financial assistance in any form for any recognized medical or social problem. And I am indicating abortion and sterilization specifically because this is a volatile and unpopular area.

The second is that Congress recognize that abortion per se is favored by no one, but that on an individual basis it does have great importance, and that this importance must be determined only within the relationship of a woman and her physician.

As a point of fact, our Supreme Court has so indicated. The third is that the Congress assist in efforts to elimi-

nate the need for abortion, by taking advantage of the fact that for the first time in the history of this country we have the opportunity to study it out in the open. It is important to recognize that the need for it is a symptom of much deeper problems as a rule.

The last recommendation is that rather than withdrawing funding for study as well as treatment in this sensitive area, I would like to suggest that expanding the availability of public education, family planning, crisis intervention, individual and family counseling, would certainly be of much greater benefit to the greatest number of people.

I thank you very much.

[The following was submitted by Dr. Barr:]
EPOC CLINIC,
Winter Park,
Fla., May 31, 1974.

JOHN M. MARTIN, JR.,
Chief Counsel, Committee on Ways and Means,
Washington, D.C.

DEAR MR. MARTIN: *The following is a summary of statements to be presented by oral testimony, as requested, in 150 copies: For June 7, 1974.*

I would like to thank the Committee on Ways and Means for the opportunity of appearing and speaking against any efforts to eliminate needed governmental assistance from the assistance of any medical problem in general, and those of abortion and family planning in particular. I make this plea in the name of your extending the most good to that segment of our population needing help in these matters.

Let me ask you to differentiate the real issue at hand. The first involves the position of Congress regarding any compelling desire to practice medicine by deciding what is or is not good medicine and enforcing those decisions by funding or denial of funding to broad segments of population dependent upon governmental assistance for medical care. You do have the power, but I am in strong hopes that you do not have the wish to maintain that posture. I am not speaking down to you as a specialist in gynecology to laymen. I am appealing to you not to make mass judgments, most especially when good judgments must be made on individual bases.

The second involves an objective view of legalized abortion and family planning per se. The most conservative and even reactionary segments of the medical and social professions have endorsed legalized abortion simply from a recognition of need. Dire, pressing, catastrophic need, on individual bases. Need that has led hundreds of thousands of women unable to cope with an unwanted pregnancy to knowingly risk serious injury and death in the absence of legalization. Needs predicated upon cases involving survival of a family unit, cancer, emotional stress, rape, teenage pregnancy, etc., are obvious. There are many more subtle associations with equally severe need.

I will dismiss as nonsense the premise that you have heard that anyone ... patient, physician, social worker, clergyman, takes abortion lightly. I further dismiss as nonsense the premise that anyone "favors abortion." Believe me that no one "favors" abortion or has anything good to say about it except that for those in need it may save or make possible the survival of a woman's or a family's physical, emotional, or social well being. And that is the name of good medicine, from personal to state levels.

The third issue involves the political pressures put upon you by vociferous and well financed individuals and groups, hoping to force you into forgetting the first two. With false morality devoid of compassion, with self-righteousness placing their own psychological needs above the real day to day needs of others, without understanding or wanting to understand the real problems of those in need, the anti-abortion individuals and groups have demanded that you give them self satisfaction at the expense of whoever else may suffer in the process. On this point I plead that you do not yield!

Preventing the imposition of the philosophies of a pow-

erful few upon the many is reflected in our government in precedents all the way from separation of church and state to antitrust legislation. I plead with you not to violate that basic premise.

The fourth issue is that of economics, the most significant to the named function of this Committee, but the least significant overall. The economics of not forcing unwanted pregnancy upon the indigent [or anyone else for that matter] by far outweigh those of doing so, on a personal, family, state, and national level.

Permit me to make the following recommendations:

(1) That the Congress not disallow medical financial assistance in any form for abortion or any other recognized medical or social problem.

(2) That the Congress recognize that abortion per se is "favored" by no one, but that the need for it has, does, and shall exist on individual bases, and that those bases must be determined only within the relationship of a woman and her physician.

(3) That the Congress assist in efforts to eliminate the need for abortion by recognizing it as a frequent symptom of deeper medical-social problems. We have the first opportunity in the history of this country to study the problems openly and approach them with medical competency. Any repressive action would be detrimental to the welfare of present and future generations.

(4) That funding for study as well as treatment should not be withdrawn but developed, incorporating services of public education, expanded family planning, crisis intervention, individual and family counseling. I have a personal commitment to pursue this goal and would be happy to expand upon the particulars if requested. With this view, permit me to suggest that the Congress may assume the enlightened posture of constructive action, analogous to no less than bringing the mentally ill out of the cellars many generations ago.

Thank you again for your interest, and for the opportunity of appearing before you.

SAMUEL J. BARR, M.D.

Mr. BURKE. Do you run a clinic, Doctor?

Dr. BARR. Yes, I do.

Mr. BURKE. Is it an abortion clinic?

Dr. BARR. That is correct. It is in Winter Park, Fla. I have a private practice of gynecology but I opened this clinic to provide the needs of that area. It has been open a year and I have had a chance to learn a great deal about the problems by directing it.

Mr. BURKE. How many abortions were performed at your clinic last year?

Dr. BARR. About 4,000.

Mr. BURKE. What do you charge for an abortion?

Dr. BARR. The complete cost that we have is $175 as an outpatient. This includes not only the procedure but individual counseling by degreed social workers, which we feel is very important to rule out any problems indicating that the abortion would not be valuable.

It also includes the laboratory workup tantamount to anything available in full hospital setting, and overall the services compare with what would otherwise cost the patient approximately $500 or much more if obtained in a hospital setting. This is an outpatient facility.

Mr. BURKE. Does that complete your testimony, Doctor?

Dr. BARR. Yes, sir.

Appendix E: *Who Supports and Who Opposes Legal Abortion?*

Who supports and who opposes legal abortion? Where does the American Medical Association stand? The John Birch Society and the Ku Klux Klan? The Baptist and Methodist churches?

The following list gives those who support and oppose legal abortion in each area of our society. Even a moment's attention offers many familiar names, and quite a few surprises. A representative sample of polls is also included.

Organizations Supporting the Right to Choose	**Organizations Against Abortion**
Legal	*Legal*
American Bar Association American Civil Liberties Union National Emergency Civil Liberties Committee New York Women's Bar Association	
Medical	*Medical*
American Association of Planned Parenthood Physicians American College of Obstetricians and Gynecologists American College of Osteopathic Obstetricians and Gynecologists American Medical Association American Medical Women's Association American Psychiatric Association American Psychoanalytic Association American Public Health Association Group for the Advancement of Psychiatry Medical Committee for Human Rights National Council of Obstetrics and Gynecology National Medical Association	American Association of Pro-Life Obstetricians and Gynecologists California Medical Association Catholic Hospitals Associations/World-wide Doctors and Nurses Against Abortion Doctors and Nurses for Life Massachusetts Medical Society National Nurses for Life Scientists for Life

Organizations Supporting the Right to Choose	**Organizations Against Abortion**

Medical

Physicians Forum
Student American Medical
    Association
Womens Medical Association

Medical

Social Service

American Friends Service
    Committee
American Psychological
    Association
Association for Voluntary
    Sterilization
Family Service Association
Federation of Protestant
    Welfare Agencies
National Association of
    Social Workers
National Committee for
    Children and Youth
National Council on Family
    Relations
National Welfare Rights
    Organization
Planned Parenthood-World
    Population
President's Task Force on the
    Mentally Handicapped
White House Conference on
    Children and Youth

Social Service

Birth Right

Religious

American Baptist Churches
    in the USA

Religious

Cardinal Mindszenty
    Foundation

Organizations Supporting the Right to Choose	*Organizations Against Abortion*
Religious	*Religious*
American Ethical Union	Christians Against Abortion
American Humanist Association	Christian Crusade (Billey Jean Hargiss)
American Jewish Congress	Lutheran Synod
American Lutheran Church, Exec. Committee of the Comm. on Church and Society	National Board for Social Concern of the Lutheran Church
American Protestant Hospital Association	Rabbinical Council of America
Baptist Joint Committee on Public Affairs	Roman Catholic Conference of Bishops
B'nai B'rith	Society for the Christian Commonwealth
Catholics for a Free Choice	The Catholic Church
Central Conference of American Rabbis	The Church of Jesus Christ of Latter Day Saints (Mormons)
Church of the Brethren	
Church Women United, Board of Managers	
Clergy Consultation Service on Abortion	
Ecumenical Foundation for Higher Education (Campus Clergy)	
Episcopal Churchwomen of the USA	
Federation of Jewish Philanthropies	
Friends Committee on National Legislation	
Lutheran Church in America	
Moravian Church, Northern Province Synod	

Organizations Supporting the Right to Choose	***Organizations Against Abortion***
Religious	*Religious*

Religious

National Association for the
  Laity
National Council of Jewish
  Women
National Federation of
  Temple Sisterhoods
Presbyterian Church in U.S.
Religious Affairs Committee
  of Planned Parenthood/
  World of Population
Religious Coalition for
  Abortion Rights
Unitarian Universalist
  Association
Unitarian Universalist
  Women's Federation
United Church of Canada,
  General Council
United Church of Christ
United Methodist Church
United Methodist Church,
  Women's Division
Union of American Hebrew
  Congregations
United Presbyterian Church
  USA
Women's League for Con-
  servative Judaism
Women's Program Unit,
  United Presbyterian
  Church USA
United Synagogue of America
Young Women's Christian
  Association

Organizations Supporting the Right to Choose	Organizations Against Abortion

Women

American Association of University Women
Fiftieth Anniversary Conference of the Women's Bureau of the US Dept. of Labor
National Council of Women of the US
National Organization for Women
National Women's Lobby, Inc.
National Women's Political Caucus
Women's Equity Action League
Women's National Abortion Action Coalition

Women

Feminists for Life
Happiness of Womanhood (HOW)
Stop ERA
Women Concerned for the Unborn Child

Other

American Association of United Nations
Americans for Democratic Action
American Home Economics Association
Americans United for Separation of Church and State
Citizens Advisory Council on the Status of Women
Coalition of Concerned Black Americans
Consumer Action Now

Other

Ad Hoc Committee
Americans Against Abortion
American Conservative Union
American Party (Formerly American Independent Party)
AWARE
Campus Crusade
Committee of 10 Million
John Birch Society
Ku Klux Klan
Liberty Lobby

Organizations Supporting the Right to Choose	*Organizations Against Abortion*
Other	*Other*

Environmental Policy Center
Federation of American
Scientists
Friends of the Earth
Izaak Walton League
Junior League
National Abortion Rights
Action League
National Council of Negro
Women
National Conference of Com-
missioners on Uniform
State Laws
Population Association of
America
Sierra Club
Society for the Psychological
Study of Social Issues
Union 1199 (Hospital and
Health Care Workers)
United Automobile Workers
Union
Urban Coalition
Workmens Circle
Zero Population Growth, Inc.

National Association of Pro
America
National Pro-Life Info.
Service
National Right to Life
Committee
National States Rights Party
National Youth–Pro-Life
(Life Action Committee)
Pro-Life Weekly
Project Lifeguard (Society for
Christian Commonwealth)
Student Coalition for the
Human Life Amendment
Teen Challenge
The Navigators
U.N. Coalition for Life
Volcum (Value of Life
Committee)
We, the People!
Young Americans for
Freedom (YAF)
Youth Coalition Against
Abortion (YAF)

**Public Opinion Polls Since The Supreme Court
Decisions of 1973
(compiled September 1976)**

NEW YORK TIMES/CBS NEWS POLL—September 5, 1976
—random selection of 1,703 registered voters. (NY Times/CBS
News, 1976)

"Do you favor an amendment to the Constitution that would make abortions illegal, or do you oppose such a change in the law?"

Favor	Oppose	Don't Know/ No Answer
32%	56%	12%

Respondents who were in favor of an amendment supported:

    Carter—47%   Ford—30%   Others—23%

Respondents who were not in favor of an amendment supported:

    Carter—45%   Ford—35%   Others—20%

HARRIS SURVEY—Spring 1972, 1973, 1975, 1976—interviews with 1,000 to 2,000 adults nationwide. (Louis Harris and Associates, Inc., 1972–1976)

"Do you favor or oppose the U.S. Supreme Court decision making abortions up to three months of pregnancy legal?"

	1972*	1973	1975	1976†
Favor	42%	52%	54%	54%
Oppose	46	41	38	39
Not sure	12	7	8	7

* The question for the 1972 survey did not make reference to the 1973 Supreme Court decisions, but asked if abortion up to three months of pregnancy should be legal.

† In 1976, the Harris Survey asked a cross section of 1,512 nationwide: "In 1973, the U.S. Supreme Court decided that state laws making it illegal for a woman to have an abortion up to three months of pregnancy were unconstitutional, and that the decision on whether a woman should have an abortion up to three months of pregnancy should be left up to the woman and her doctor. In general, do you favor or oppose the U.S. Supreme

Court decision making abortions up to three months of pregnancy legal?"

GALLUP POLL—March 1976—personal interviews with 1,525 adults nationwide (Field Enterprises, Inc., 1976)
"A constitutional amendment has been proposed which would prohibit abortions, except when the pregnant woman's life is in danger. Would you favor this amendment which would prohibit abortions or would you oppose it?"

	Favor	*Oppose*	*No Opinion*
National	45%	49%	6%
College background	30	65	5
High school	49	46	5
Grade school	56	31	13

GALLUP POLL—April 1975—interviews with 1,535 persons 18 or older nationwide. (Field Enterprises, Inc., 1975)
"Do you think that abortion should be legal under any circumstances, legal under certain circumstances, or illegal in all circumstances?"

Should be legal under any circumstances	21%
Should be legal only under certain circumstances	54
Should be illegal in all circumstances	22
No opinion	3

NATIONAL OBSERVER PLEBISCITE—February 22–March 5, 1976, page one ballot of three choices offered to readers nationwide, to which 13,572 responded. (Reflects intensity of feeling on issue.) (*National Observer*, 1976)

71% or 9,683 agreed: "let the Supreme Court decision legalizing abortion stand."
23.9% or 3,247 agreed: "amend the Constitution to outlaw all abortions."

4.7% or 642 agreed: "amend the Constitution to return abortion matters to the states."

NBC NEWS POLL—February 26–28, 1976—interviews with 1,500 adults throughout the United States. (NBC News, 1976)
"Are you in favor of an Amendment to the Constitution which would make it illegal to have an abortion or would you oppose such an Amendment?"

Opposed	In Favor	Not Sure
66%	26%	8%

NEW YORK TIMES/CBS NEWS POLL—February 2–8, 1976 —interviews with 1,463 adult men and women across the continental United States. (NY Times/CBS News, 1976)
"The right of a woman to have an abortion should be left entirely up to the woman and her doctor."

Agree	Disagree	Don't Know
67%	26%	7%

KNIGHT-RIDDER NEWSPAPERS SURVEY—January 12–17, 1976—interviews with 1,117 adults in 21 cities. (Knight-Ridder Newspapers, 1976)
"If a woman wants to have an abortion, that is a matter for her and her doctor to decide and the government should have nothing to do with it."

Agree	Disagree	Not Sure
81%	15%	4%

Agreement by Religion:
Protestants—82%   Jews—98%   Catholics—76%

NBC NEWS POLL—November 6, 1974—interviews with a national probability sample of 9,733 voters; January 4, 1976—telephone interviews, nationwide, with 2,836 adults. (NBC News, 1974, 1976)
"Would you like to see abortion laws changed so that it

would be harder for a woman to get an abortion, easier for a woman to get an abortion, or do you think abortion laws should be left the way they are?"

| | 1974 | | | | | 1976 |
	East	Midwest	South	West	Nation	Nation
Harder	30%	36%	33%	28%	32%	33%
No change	31	28	27	27	28	32
Easier	30	25	27	37	30	24
Not sure	9	11	13	8	10	11

WASHINGTON SURVEY—February and April 1975—interviews with an area probability sample of 2,102 residents of Greater Washington, D.C. (Bureau of Social Science Research, Inc., 1975)

"The decision to have an abortion should be made solely by a woman and her physician."

Agree—77%   Disagree—20%   No Opinion—4%

DEVRIES POLL—December 1974—interviews with 4,004 adults nationwide. Commissioned by the National Committee for a Human Life Amendment. (DeVries and Associates, March, 1975)

"Abortion should not be allowed under any circumstances."

	Total	Catholic	Protestant	Jewish
Strongly agree	15.8%	22.3%	14.6%	2.6%
Mildly agree	7.8	9.0	7.9	3.6
Mildly disagree	21.7	22.7	23.2	4.5
Strongly disagree	50.5	42.0	49.5	86.9
Not sure	4.2	4.0	4.8	2.4

VIRGINIA SLIMS AMERICAN WOMEN'S OPINION POLL—Spring 1974—interviews with 3,006 women and 1,002 men. (The Roper Organization, Inc., 1974)

"Laws making abortion legal should be repealed."

	Agree	*Disagree*	*Not Sure*
Women	36%	50%	14%
Men	31	55	14

"Where abortions are legal, the decision about an abortion should be left up to a woman and her doctor."

	Agree	*Disagree*	*Not Sure*
Women	74%	15%	12%
Men	70	17	13

NATIONAL OPINION RESEARCH SURVEY—July 1972 & July 1973—interviews with a national probability sample of men and women (quota sample at block level). Commissioned by the *National Catholic Reporter*. (National Opinion Research Center, 1972, 1973)

Attitudes Toward Abortion by Religious Affiliation (Per Cent Approve)

Reason for Abortion	Protestant		Catholic		Jew	
	1972	1973	1972	1973	1972	1973
Danger to mother's health	83%	91%	80%	88%	96%	100%
Rape	74	81	70	75	96	98
Chance of defective child	75	83	67	77	91	100
Does not want more children	36	46	29	34	70	91
Mother is unwed	39	48	32	34	80	88
Too poor to have more children	45	52	36	39	78	92

CONGRESSIONAL POLLS—93 constituent polls taken during the 93rd Congress included a question on abortion. Although the wording of the questions varied so that direct comparison of the polls is not possible, 73 polls showed majority support of the right to abortion, 2 polls showed majority support of states' rights, 13 polls showed no majority, and only

5 polls showed majority opposition to the right to choose abortion in the Member's district.

Appendix F: *Drugs That Cause Fetal Problems and Malformations*

The drug thalidomide brought into sharp focus the fact that certain medications might be safe for the mother but might cause problems with a fetus if taken early in pregnancy. Very few drugs cause problems as dramatic as thalidomide, which led to improper development of arms and legs. Most medications *are* safe, even when they are taken in the early stages of pregnancy. But all medications should be known by name, and the woman who suspects that she might be pregnant should have the opportunity to check with this *basic, not total* list of possible problem drugs to reassure herself and seek medical advice immediately.

Certain drugs have a proven capacity to cause various kinds of fetal defects. The largest group in this category are drugs used against cancer. They are called antineoplastic agents, and the following is a list of specific ones which may cause fetal deformity:

Aminopterin	Colchicine
Busulfan (Myleran)	Cytoxan
Chlorambucil (Leukeran)	Mercaptopurine
	Methotrexate

Thalidomide can cause defects of arms and legs. It has never been used much in the United States, and was originally prescribed as a sleeping tablet. In all probability it will never again be sold in this country.

Significant doses of a form of estrogen, diethylstilbestrol, had been prescribed many years ago for bleeding problems in early pregnancy. Cases have been reported of fibrous degeneration and even carcinoma in females whose mothers had been given this drug early in pregnancy. The medication is no longer used for this purpose.

Radioactive iodine in significant doses can lead to impaired thyroid function in the newborn if the mother receives it during pregnancy. Before taking any radioactive material for treatment or diagnosis, women and their physicians should always check for the possibility of an ongoing pregnancy.

Birth control pills themselves are occasionally continued early in pregnancy during those rare instances in which a pregnancy has occurred despite their use. In those instances, the pills can act as male hormones in having a masculinizing effect upon possible female fetuses. The practical importance of this information is that women taking the pill must report any irregularity of usage and even any skipping of periods until all question of pregnancy is resolved.

There are other drugs suspected of causing fetal defects, most especially if used in high doses over prolonged periods of time. Commonly recognized agents include large doses of alcohol; hormones, including steroids; Dexedrine (dextroamphetamine), as in preparations for weight control; quinine; Reserpine; streptomycin; tetracyclines; vitamin D; warfarin; and significant exposure to X-rays. The amount of radiation received should be checked with a radiologist if it occurred during an unsuspected pregnancy. Most short diagnostic studies would not constitute a real threat to a pregnancy. Extensive procedures, such as lower bowel studies, may. A professional opinion must be sought on the basis of the actual exposure in any particular case, and no across-the-board generalities must be accepted.

Many other drugs are being studied continuously for the possibility of causing birth defects, although there is as yet no definitive evidence that they do. Among these are commonly recognized preparations including aspirin, Librium, Miltown (or Equanil), Preludin, and LSD. Laboratory animals have demonstrated chromosomal damage with LSD usage, but inconclusive evidence exists concerning its effects on humans. Certainly, exposure to high, prolonged doses of LSD is cause for worry for many reasons, but in the absence of other grounds, it would be difficult to justify abortion for this reason alone.

Revised lists of the status of drugs and their side effects are published continuously and any woman suspecting that she might be pregnant should check with her doctor concerning possible ill effects of her medications on the pregnancy. One important contribution toward helping women safeguard themselves would be the requirement that *all prescriptions have their contents listed on the label*. Many physicians have this done routinely for a variety of good reasons. Concern for possible effects during pregnancy is simply one more.

Appendix G: *Statistics of IUD Failures*

Over a three-year period 15,000 consecutive requests for abortion were studied at EPOC Clinic to determine the needs which arose from IUD failures. A total of 125 such cases were noted, indicating 0.83 percent cause. The results may well be a biostatistician's nightmare because it is virtually impossible to correlate the failures with the actual numbers of IUD's inserted and working, with a breakdown by type, or with the relative skills of the physicians performing insertions. Only six months into the study the FDA advised all physicians not to prescribe the Dalkon Shield because of possible complications of septic abortion in cases of pregnancy occurring with the shield still in place. It was withdrawn from the market one fifth of the way through our survey, though most women who had it inserted continued to wear it. On the other hand, the Copper Seven did not make an appearance until halfway through the study, and so the low numbers of its failures must be interpreted as low usage rates rather than a relatively great success rate. By the same token this fact must be considered in reviewing its relatively short retention percentages.

An additional factor is that the Lippes Loop and Saf-T-Coil were available years before the Dalkon Shield, but for a comparative two-year span of 1971–72 the shield outsold the loop and coil by about 63 to 37 percent.

All of these points must be stated because many variables

prevent the assertion of hard conclusions. Nevertheless, the study has validity because it tells what actually happened. It might have been professionally "safer" to suppress or discard these findings. But then, unless factual information is presented, not even the experts are given much help. Our findings appear in the following table:

Intrauterine device	Dalkon Shield	Saf-T-Coil	Lippes Loop	Copper Seven
Total numbers of failures	44	40	26	15
Percent of total numbers	35.2	32	20.8	12
Total months of usage before failure	822	540	586	161
Retention Average months	18.7	13.5	22.5	10.7
Retention 12 months or less	56.8%	62%	58%	73%
Retention 13–24 months	22.7%	33%	15%	27%
Retention Over 24 months	20.5%	5%	27%	0%

All of the cases tabulated represent intrauterine devices removed in the clinic in the course of suction curettage. Most of them were located in the lower uterine segment near the endocervical os. No extra difficulty and no excessive bleeding was encountered because of the presence of an IUD. Only one case was encountered in which an IUD was identified by X-ray as being in the abdominal cavity before any procedure was performed.

The patient was hospitalized, and under the same anesthetic, suction curettage was used to terminate the pregnancy, and then the IUD was removed with grasping forceps, using the laparoscope. It had become adherent to the anterior abdominal wall peritoneum with fine adhesions.

My personal choice of an IUD is the Lippes Loop. It seems to have provided the best overall results with the least number of problems. Furthermore, I am not convinced that copper wrappings offer anything close to the last word in IUD contraception. I feel that too many failures have occurred in the relatively short time of its availability, compared to the Lippes Loop, for example. I have had no observations of progesterone-like compounds contained in an intrauterine device, the newest arrival on the scene. Whether the idea works well or not in practice remains to be seen. One defect inherent in the IUD is the increasing number of women who find themselves with an unwanted pregnancy because their doctors thought it a "good idea" to remove the IUD for "a rest" to the uterus, with or without valid reason.

Let me add a final note in still one more area of controversy. The policy of my clinic is *not* to recommend abortion on the *exclusive* grounds of an IUD's being present with an ongoing pregnancy. Granted, allowing the pregnancy to continue does carry increased risk of serious infection, which may destroy the pregnancy and harm the mother as well. Most of the time, there is no great problem in decision because of the many factors which had led the woman to use this long-term contraceptive in the first place. If those other factors weigh heavily in favor of abortion, then the risk of infection is just one more consideration on the scales. But the woman who has been fairly advised of this risk, and wants the pregnancy enough to assume it, should not be pressed into abortion, in my opinion. The IUD itself cannot harm the fetus because it must be located outside of the amniotic sac, and it has been shown many times over that a trouble-free pregnancy may result, with the IUD's being passed out with the placenta at delivery. Once again, it is the woman's own informed choice that must be respected.

Appendix H: *The History and Current Status of Abortion*

The History of Abortion

During almost all of civilization's history abortion has been considered a proper procedure. Records indicate that it was commonly practiced in Egypt and in China thousands of years before Christ. It was also practiced freely in the Greek city-states and Rome. Ancient religions did not bar abortion as such, but what prosecution did exist seems to have been based upon a concept of violating a father's right to his offspring. About 400 years B.C., Hippocrates framed his famous oath, which, among other things, spoke against abortion and suicide. Most Greek thinkers, on the other hand, such as Plato and Aristotle, spoke in favor of abortion, at least prior to viability.

In British common law, from the thirteenth century onward, abortion performed before "quickening"—the first recognizable movement of the fetus in the uterus, usually from the sixteenth to eighteenth week of pregnancy—was not considered an offense. Christian theology at the time held that the fetus became animated by a rational soul and abortion was therefore a serious crime only at forty days after conception for a boy and eighty days for a girl. This position was interesting since no method of sex determination was specified. In the United States the common law ideas of England were carried over, and our founding fathers did not write abortion into the laws as a crime.

For more than 1,800 years the Catholic Church accepted abortions that were performed before quickening. Only a century ago, in 1869, the Catholic Church took the position that all abortion was to be considered murder. During the 1800s, antiabortion laws sprang up in England and the United States, but most of these carried the exception of the necessity of saving the life of the woman.

There were several reasons why antiabortion laws came

into effect. The first was concerned with the health of the mother in the absence of antisepsis, antibiotics, and adequate medical techniques. In the mid-1800s all surgery was extremely dangerous and carried a high rate of morbidity and mortality. All surgery was considered best discouraged.

The next reason had to do with the simple concept that in numbers there is strength. In the Catholic countries of Europe, any and all measures that might limit population growth, ranging from contraception to abortion, were condemned. In the United States and England, the demands of industry for workers carried the same implication, the need for more people, as many people as possible. The ravaging effects of our civil war plus expansions into the western territories also echoed the demands for "more people!"

Last but not least, the middle of the last century saw a prolonged surfacing of the related ideas that sex for pleasure was bad, that pregnancy was punishment for pleasure, and that fear of pregnancy would reinforce morals. The law even banned from the mails any literature, medicine, or article to do with contraception or abortion.

Scandinavian countries, on the other hand, liberalized definitions of need for abortion. This was also done in most East European countries, including Russia and Poland.

Japan arrived at legal abortion as a matter of national necessity. What with returning troops after World War II, a devastated economy, and a baby boom resulting from wartime nationalism, the country was in an economic bind. The Eugenic Protection Law instituted abortion as the national method of population control.

In England, the Infant Life Preservation Act of 1929 emphasized the concept of viability by naming as a crime the destruction of the life of a child capable of being born alive unless preserving the life of the mother was a factor. A further step was taken in the Abortion Act of 1967, which permitted abortion if the continuation of the pregnancy would involve risks to the life of the pregnant woman, or any existing children of her family, greater than if the pregnancy were terminated, or if there was substantial risk that if the child were born it would suffer from such physical or mental abnormalities as to be seriously handicapped.

Back in the United States, public opinion pressed for abortion reform and the first significant step in this direction was the proposal of a model penal code by the American Law Institute in 1959. This included provisions that a licensed physician could legally terminate a pregnancy if he or she believed that it threatened the life or would greatly impair the physical or mental health of the mother; if the child would be born with grave physical or mental defects; or if the pregnancy resulted from rape or incest. In 1962, the great thalidomide tragedies further emphasized the problem when a woman who had taken this drug was denied abortion in Arizona, her native state, and had to travel to Sweden to obtain it. There, evidence verified fetal deformity. Other dramatic cases came to light. A woman mental patient became pregnant after having been raped by an inmate who had escaped from maximum-security quarters. A New York couple was refused abortion despite the woman's having German measles in the first trimester. The child was born deaf, blind, mentally retarded, spastic, and with a defective heart.

By 1970, Alaska, Hawaii, New York, and Washington legalized all abortions performed by physicians up to a certain point in pregnancy. The American Bar Association approved a uniform abortion act as model legislation, indicating that neither husband's nor parental consent should be required. Finally, in 1973, the United States Supreme Court interpreted the status of abortion under the right of privacy as guaranteed under the Fourteenth Amendment of the Constitution.

The Current Status of Abortion

The amount of information coming to light since legalization has been most revealing. Before that time it was impossible to get an accurate picture of true conditions other than by studying septic hospital wards of large hospitals and scanning police blotters, which record severe injury. It has been estimated, though, that some nine hundred thousand women a year received back-alley abortions prior to legalization in 1973. Since that historic decision, so much statistical data has become available that it is impossible to present it all. The following is a summary of its high points.

One estimate showed that seven out of ten legal abortions performed in 1974 would have taken place illegally if abortion were outlawed. During the first year following legalization, there was a 40 percent drop in abortion-related deaths.

Abortions performed during the first trimester of pregnancy are six times safer than childbirth. The statistical preponderance of women requesting termination of pregnancy in the second trimester points to the young, the poor, those living in rural areas, and those who have learned that they are carrying defective fetuses with genetic defects through medical testing that is possible only in the second trimester.

The first great study of national statistics was reported by the Center for Disease Control after analyzing data of the year 1974 from all fifty states. The data may well reflect less than the actual picture since not all abortions are reported, even with legalization. At that time two hundred and forty-two abortions per one thousand live births were reported, which represented nearly one legal abortion for every four live births.

The average statistics for women obtaining legal abortion nationwide varied slightly from those found in EPOC Clinic, but in the main they tended to be young, white, and unmarried, with low numbers of previous pregnancies and at a relatively early stage of pregnancy at the time of the procedure. About one third of the women were age nineteen or younger, a third were twenty-five years of age or older. About 70 percent were white and 30 percent were black, about 27 percent were married and 73 percent were unmarried. Close to half the women had no living children at the time of the procedure. About one fifth had one living child and about one seventh had two living children. About a fifth of all patients had three or more living children. Eighty-seven percent of the women underwent abortion during the first twelve weeks of gestation, calculated from last menstrual period.

Deaths related to abortion continued to decline since the onset of legalization. In 1974 there were twenty-four such deaths in the course of legally induced abortion. There were six deaths resulting from illegal procedures and eighteen from spontaneous abortion or, as it is commonly called, miscarriage. The death rate for legal abortion therefore was 3.1 deaths per hundred thousand abortions.

Overall, legal abortion was judged to be a safe procedure since fewer than 1 percent of all cases sustained any major complication. A frequently quoted point of perspective is that the overall incidence of abortion has come to be greater than that of tonsillectomy and the overall complication problems have come to be less.

Across the country approximately 10 percent of women requiring abortion have had repeat procedures for a variety of reasons. The range of incidence has varied by state from approximately 3 percent in Nebraska to over 20 percent in the District of Columbia and New York.

On a worldwide basis it is estimated that between 30 and 55 million abortions are induced every year. Over the past decade more than a dozen countries have made significant changes in the direction of lessening restrictions and providing full legalization. A country whose opposition to abortion has been deeply entrenched is rapidly moving toward legalization.

Four Eastern European countries have moved in the opposite direction. At the present time, about one third of the world's people live in countries with moderately restrictive laws, and a third live where abortion is either completely illegal or allowed only if the woman's life or health is severely threatened by continuation of a pregnancy. The same general problems exist for women applying for second-trimester abortion on a worldwide basis, as has been discussed in the United States. A review of world conditions has shown that the overall incidence of complications, including mortality, has dramatically declined as the availability of abortion has shifted from an illegal to a legal status, with concurrent availability of proper medical care. To date, some sixty handicapping conditions in the fetus can now be recognized during pregnancy with diagnostic tests early in the second trimester.

For those interested in greater statistical details, three sources are suggested: Planned Parenthood–World Population in New York, National Abortion Rights Action League and the Religious Coalition for Abortion Rights in Washington, D.C., and the Center for Disease Control Abortion Surveillance, published by the U.S. Department of Health, Education, and Welfare in Atlanta, Georgia. The most notable single contributor to the biostatistics of abortion is Christopher Tietze of the Population Council in New York.

Statistical Profile of 20,000 Patients Seen at EPOC Clinic

Florida, like California, has become one of the great "melting-pot" areas. Individuals and families from across the nation come to settle daily in this semitropical land of three seasons. A study of this area is not just a reflection of local color. It is a broad brushstroke of people from many states with many different backgrounds.

The greatest majority of young patients are in school. The middle and older age groups represent a relatively stable population with steady job income. Medicaid patients make up only 6.7 percent of our patients.

The median of all patients reflects the middle to upper-middle strata of all the people in this country. Every type of job description, from entertainer to stockbroker, from secretary to female firefighter, has been represented. There have been migrant farm workers, living a hand-to-mouth existence, and vastly greater numbers of wives and daughters of physicians, attorneys, engineers, and public officials of all sorts.

The most interesting thing about this vast panorama of people is not what separates them into one category or another, but the fact that they all relate to the same basic problems. It is the insignificant amount of difference from the wealthy to the poor, from the well-educated to the high school dropout, that makes the greatest impression. The couple with a $20,000 income maintaining a $40,000 mortgage and supporting two children in college may feel no more secure than a family earning half the income with half the obligations. Educational level makes no distinction in cases of IUD failures, social rape, or the intent of abstinence. Economic status melts into common denominators for the many women who feel that they have had their families and have come to a point in life where they want to establish their own identity. The only generality that applies with validity to all women is that the impact of pregnancy is both deep and real.

Note that statistics on age, race, religion, reasons for having an abortion, and referral have already been presented in Appendix A.

CONTRACEPTION

Prior contraceptive used:

73.2%	None
6.0	Pill
2.0	IUD
8.2	Foam
1.6	Diaphragm
5.4	Condom
2.6	Rhythm
0.5	Withdrawal
0.3	Sterilization
26.8	Total using contraceptives

This statistic indicates the method of birth control that was in use at the time of conception. The high percentage of women who were not using contraceptives reflects two things: First is the youth of most of the women who need abortion. Second is the simple truth that a woman who is not on contraceptives runs a high risk of an unwanted pregnancy.

One interesting phenomenon occurred during the Arab oil embargo. At this time an additional 10 percent of patients rapidly began using some method of birth control.

Planned future contraception:

92.8% Total planned future contraception
76.1 Pill
 6.9 IUD
 3.4 Sterilization
 7.1 None
 6.3 All other birth control methods

Women who have had an abortion are most eager to begin using the pill. After the shock and trauma of an unwanted pregnancy, most women want to use the most effective form of birth control available, and that is the pill. At this moment in their lives, they prefer to chance the slight risks from the pill to the dangers and pain of an unwanted pregnancy. Nearly 93 percent of all patients plan to use some sort of birth control in the future.

The Medical Profile

How Safe Is Abortion? The Actual Record: Out of twenty thousand patients, we have had the following complications. Seven patients required hospitalization for a D&C because of excessive bleeding secondary to the presence of retained tissue following abortion. These patients had sought assistance from their private physicians. Twelve patients required repeat suction curettage, performed in the clinic, for the same reason. There were six cases of postabortal endometritis, two of which required hospital observation. One patient required a laparotomy because of a severely retroverted uterus, which had been perforated. The endometrial cavity in that case was evacuated with direct visualization. Another patient did require hysterectomy because of perforation, and a third woman had a tear of endocervical tissue with secondary bleeding leading to a retroperitoneal hematoma. This was evacuated surgically without the necessity of performing a hysterectomy. Five patients continued with viable pregnancies after the suction curettage procedure in the clinic. Of these, three had second-trimester abortions at hospital facilities and two elected to keep the pregnancy. In both of the latter instances there were no reported defects in the delivered baby. It is noteworthy that in one of these two cases the pathology report of tissue submitted by the clinic from suction curettage indicated tissue compatible with the termination of a pregnancy. This patient did have a bicornate uterus. The remaining patients did rather well.

The Venereal Disease Study: We have concluded that the venereal disease rate in women presenting themselves for termination of pregnancy is as low or lower than those in the general population. This is not a firm conclusion because we lack public health data concerning the incidence of venereal disease in sexually active females, which are the sole province of our figures.

The syphilis incidence demonstrated by positive serology in the clinic was 0.02 percent. The positive incidence reported by the Health Department was 0.027 percent. The Health Department figure is for the total population of adult males, females, and children of all ages.

The clinic's incidence of positive cultures for gonorrhea by the transgrow medium technique indicated 1.42 percent. Health Department statistics for the same geographic area indicated a gonorrhea rate of 0.6 percent, but this figure reflects the total population rather than just sexually active females.

First-/Second-trimester Requests:

70.7%	Under twelve weeks
17.1	Over twelve weeks
12.2	Not pregnant

Pregnancy Order: When Do Abortions Occur in the Sequence of Childbearing?

52.0%	Multigravid patient
47.9	Primigravid patient

10.5%	Spontaneous abortions, prior medical history
11.2	Induced abortions, prior medical history
4.5	EPOC Clinic-induced abortions

Primigravidous refers to the first pregnancy. Multigravidous refers to those after the first. The term *spontaneous abortion* is the general term *miscarriage*.

Induced abortion indicates therapeutic termination of pregnancy. The surprisingly large percentages of repeat requests for termination of pregnancy raise the question of whether or not abortion is becoming popular as a form of birth control. The answer is very clear. It most certainly is not. The expense and stress of a surgical procedure of any kind removes this from the realm of possibility. All the reasons for repeat abortions are not known, but patterns are emerging that suggest these are subconscious cries for help.

Appendix I: *Why Did the Supreme Court Legalize Abortion?*

Jane Roe *et al.*, Appellants, *v.* Henry Wade
January 22, 1973

(*The Court's introduction to the question:*) This Texas federal appeal and its Georgia companion ... present constitutional challenges to state criminal abortion legislation. The Texas statutes under attack here are typical of those that have been in effect in many states for approximately a century. The Georgia statutes, in contrast, have a modern cast and are a legislative product that, to an extent at least, obviously reflects the influences of recent attitudinal change, of advancing medical knowledge and techniques, and of new thinking about an old issue.

We forthwith acknowledge our awareness of the sensitive and emotional nature of the abortion controversy, of the vigorous opposing views, even among physicians, and of the deep and seemingly absolute convictions that the subject inspires. One's philosophy, one's experiences, one's exposure to the raw edges of human existence, one's religious training, one's attitudes toward life and family and their values, and the moral standards one establishes and seeks to observe are all likely to influence and to color one's thinking and conclusions about abortion.

In addition, population growth, pollution, poverty, and racial overtones tend to complicate, not simplify, the problem.

Our task, of course, is to resolve the issue by constitutional measurement free of emotion and of predilection. We seek earnestly to do this, and because we do, we have inquired into, and in this opinion place some emphasis upon, medical and medico-legal history and what that history reveals about man's attitudes toward the abortive procedure over the centuries. We bear in mind, too, Mr. Justice Holmes' admonition in his now vindicated dissent in Lochner *v.* New York, 198 U.S. 45, 76 (1905):

> It [*the Constitution*] *is made for people of fundamentally differing views, and the accident of our finding certain opinions natural and familiar or novel and even shocking ought not to conclude our judgment upon the question whether statutes embodying them conflict with the Constitution of the United States....*

(*The specific case on which the question was decided:*) Jane Roe, a single woman who was residing in Dallas County, Texas, instituted this federal action in March 1970 against the district attorney of the county. She sought a declaratory judgment that the Texas criminal abortion statutes were unconstitutional on their face, and an injunction restraining the defendant from enforcing the statutes.

Roe alleged that she was unmarried and pregnant; that she wished to terminate her pregnancy by an abortion "performed by a competent, licensed physician, under safe, clinical conditions"; that she was unable to get a "legal" abortion in Texas because her life did not appear to be threatened by the continuation of her pregnancy; and that she could not afford to travel to another jurisdiction in order to secure a legal abortion under safe conditions. She claimed that the Texas statutes were unconstitutionally vague and that they abridged her right of personal privacy, protected by the First, Fourth, Fifth, Ninth, and Fourteenth amendments. By an amendment to her complaint Roe purported to sue "on behalf of herself and all other women" similarly situated....

(The Constitutional question of anti-abortion laws:) The principal thrust of appellant's attack on the Texas statutes is that they improperly invade a right, said to be possessed by the pregnant woman, to choose to terminate her pregnancy. Appellant would discover this right in the concept of personal "liberty" embodied in the Fourteenth Amendment's Due Process Clause; or in personal, marital, familial, and sexual privacy said to be protected by the Bill of Rights or its penumbras. . . .

(Two key points from American history:) It is thus apparent that at common law, at the time of the adoption of our Constitution, and throughout the major portion of the nineteenth century, abortion was viewed with less disfavor than under most American statutes currently in effect. Phrasing it another way, a woman enjoyed a substantially broader right to terminate a pregnancy then than she does in most states today. At least with respect to the early stage of pregnancy, and very possibly without such a limitation, the opportunity to make this choice was present in this country well into the nineteenth century. Even later, the law continued for some time to treat less punitively an abortion procured in early pregnancy. . . .

The antiabortion mood prevalent in this country in the late nineteenth century was shared by the medical profession. Indeed, the attitude of the profession may have played a significant role in the enactment of stringent criminal abortion legislation during that period. . . .

(The rights and duty of the state to involve itself in regulating abortions:) The state has a legitimate interest in seeing to it that abortion, like any other medical procedure, is performed under circumstances that ensure maximum safety for the patient. This interest obviously extends at least to the performing physician and his staff, to the facilities involved, to the availability of aftercare, and to adequate provision for any complication or emergency that might arise. The prevalence of high mortality rates at illegal "abortion mills" strengthens, rather than weakens, the state's interest in regulating the con-

ditions under which abortions are performed. Moreover, the risk to the woman increases as her pregnancy continues. Thus the state retains a definite interest in protecting the woman's own health and safety when an abortion is proposed at a late stage of pregnancy.

(*The reason why the Supreme Court legalized abortion:*) This right of privacy, whether it be founded in the Fourteenth Amendment's concept of personal liberty and restrictions upon state action, as we feel it is, or, as the district court determined, in the Ninth Amendment's reservation of rights to the people, is broad enough to encompass a woman's decision whether or not to terminate her pregnancy. The detriment that the state would impose upon the pregnant woman by denying this choice altogether is apparent. Specific and direct harm medically diagnosable even in early pregnancy may be involved. Maternity, or additional offspring, may force upon the woman a distressful life and future. Psychological harm may be imminent. Mental and physical health may be taxed by child care. There is also the distress, for all concerned, associated with the unwanted child, and there is the problem of bringing a child into a family already unable, psychologically and otherwise, to care for it. In other cases, as in this one, the additional difficulties and continuing stigma of unwed motherhood may be involved. All these are factors the woman and her responsible physician necessarily will consider in consultation.

(*When does life begin?*) Texas urges that, apart from the Fourteenth Amendment, life begins at conception and is present throughout pregnancy, and that, therefore, the state has a compelling interest in protecting that life from and after conception. We need not resolve the difficult question of when life begins. When those trained in the respective disciplines of medicine, philosophy, and theology are unable to arrive at any consensus, the judiciary, at this point in the development of man's knowledge, is not in a position to speculate as to the answer.

It should be sufficient to note briefly the wide divergence of thinking on this most sensitive and difficult question. There has always been strong support for the view that life does not begin until live birth. This was the belief of the Stoics. It appears to be the predominant, though not the unanimous, attitude of the Jewish faith. It may be taken to represent also the position of a large segment of the Protestant community, insofar as that can be ascertained; organized groups that have taken a formal position on the abortion issue have generally regarded abortion as a matter for the conscience of the individual and her family.... The Aristotelian theory of "mediate animation," which held sway throughout the Middle Ages and the Renaissance in Europe, continued to be official Roman Catholic dogma until in the nineteenth century, despite opposition to this "ensoulment" theory from those in the Church who would recognize the existence of life from the moment of conception. The latter is now, of course, the official belief of the Catholic Church....

In areas other than criminal abortion the law has been reluctant to endorse any theory that life, as we recognize it, begins before live birth or to accord legal rights to the unborn except in narrowly defined situations and except when the rights are contingent upon live birth. In short, the unborn have never been recognized in the law as persons in the whole sense....

In view of all this, we do not agree that by adopting one theory of life Texas may override the rights of the pregnant woman that are at stake.

(*The Court's declaration:*) Our conclusion that Art. 1196 is unconstitutional means, of course, that the Texas abortion statutes, as a unit, must fall....

It is so ordered.

CONCLUSION

The time and tides of our history brought women a new dimension of relationships to themselves, their children, husbands, or lovers. They are reaching for self-identity, much of which revolves around the free choice of family determination. Abortion is just part of this evolution. Those who have the need deserve our care and compassion, nothing less.

Where do you fit? A while ago you may have wondered. Now I hope that you may find it is to you this book is written.

To those who love and those who have
the warmth of understanding

To those who feel that needless pain
and death are not a virtue

To those who have the courage and
the will to make life better

INDEX